Public Health Ethics

**For Louise, Reuben,
Arianne and Solomon**

Public Health Ethics

Second Edition

Stephen Holland

polity

The right of Stephen Holland to be identified as Author of this Work has been asserted in accordance with the UK Copyright, Designs and Patents Act 1988.

First published in 2007 by Polity Press

This edition published in 2015 by Polity Press

Polity Press
65 Bridge Street
Cambridge CB2 1UR, UK

Polity Press
350 Main Street
Malden, MA 02148, USA

ISBN-13: 978-0-7456-6218-3
ISBN-13: 978-0-7456-6219-0 (pb)

A catalogue record for this book is available from the British Library.

Holland, Stephen (Stephen Michael), 1963- author.
   Public health ethics / Stephen Holland. – Second edition.
      p. ; cm.
   Includes bibliographical references and index.
   ISBN 978-0-7456-6218-3 (hardback) – ISBN 0-7456-6218-8 (hardback) – ISBN 978-0-7456-6219-0 (paperback) – ISBN 0-7456-6219-6 (paperback)
   I. Title.
   [DNLM: 1. Public Health–ethics. WA 21]
   R724
   174.2'8–dc23
                                                              2014007911

Typeset in 10.5 on 12 pt Times NRMT
by Toppan Best-set Premedia Limited
Printed and bound in Great Britain by Clays Ltd, St Ives PLC.

The publisher has used its best endeavours to ensure that the URLs for external websites referred to in this book are correct and active at the time of going to press. However, the publisher has no responsibility for the websites and can make no guarantee that a site will remain live or that the content is or will remain appropriate.

Every effort has been made to trace all copyright holders, but if any have been inadvertently overlooked the publisher will be pleased to include any necessary credits in any subsequent reprint or edition.

For further information on Polity, visit our website: www.politybooks.com

Contents

Introduction |

In introducing public health ethics, it is worth explaining how it evolved out of two more established subjects, namely, medical ethics and bioethics. Medical ethics is a broad discipline in which ethical obligations in medicine and health care are analysed. It developed in response to various factors. One such factor is that medicine and health care present opportunities for enormous benefits and devastating harms because they address urgent aspects of people's lives. Another is that there has been a tendency throughout the history of medical practice and research towards insensitivity based on somewhat authoritarian attitudes. Also, post-war developments of new biomedical innovations in fields such as genetics and stem cell research have created exciting, but potentially morally hazardous, medical possibilities (Hope 2004). In the late 1960s, bioethics emerged as a branch of medical ethics. Bioethics tends to be undertaken by non-medical professionals such as philosophers and lawyers, and focuses more on the ethical implications of biotechnological advances than on patient–doctor interaction (Jonsen 1998).

Subjects such as medical ethics and bioethics are not merely academic or scholarly: they have a practical impact. Principles identified and clarified by medical ethicists, notably around respect for individual patient autonomy, have helped establish rights to such things as consent and confidentiality (Beauchamp and Childress 2013). In turn, this has altered the way medicine and health care are researched and delivered. Bioethicists have influenced the development and practice of new biomedical technologies such as stem cell therapies by, for example, analysing the moral status of human embryos (Holland 2003, 2012a). Applying findings in medical ethics and bioethics has resulted in health-related practices being ruled in and ruled out, the promotion of benefits over harms, and curbing of medical authoritarianism. And such achievements have helped engender public trust in medical research and health care delivery.

All this is by way of introducing public health ethics: public health ethics is an offshoot of medical ethics, but distinctive from bioethics because of the nature of public health itself. Although public health is hard to define, its distinctive characteristic is its population perspective (Turnock 2004). In contrast to the focus on individual patients typical of clinical medicine, public health brings into view entire populations, or sizeable subgroups within a wider population. The main aims of public health are to measure, explain, maintain and improve the health status of such target populations. Principal public health activities include describing health characteristics of communities, analysing causal factors in populations' health, and devising and implementing programmes to maintain or improve the health of the public. The emphasis in public health tends to be on preventing disease and disability, and promoting health. Public health recognizes both the multi-dimensional nature of health determinants and the complex interaction of factors (biological, social, environmental, etc.) that influence health status. Relatedly, public health tends to be a multi-agency endeavour backed by executive and legislative powers. The basis of public health is provided by empirical, quantifiable data acquired by epidemiologic research and population surveillance; although the ultimate goal of public health is to save real lives and help real people, its success is measured by statistical lives and rates of incidence of disease.

Specific types of public health activities include mass immunization campaigns, screening programmes and the various interventions loosely labelled health promotion. Two watersheds in the development of debates about the ethics of such activities are discernible, one around 1990, the other around 2000 (Faden and Kass 1991; Kass 2004). Prior to the 1990s, some medical ethicists were alert to the relevance of ethics to public health (Beauchamp 1980, 1985, 1988; Lappé 1983, 1985, 1986; cf. Kass 2004: 235–6). And some public health activities occasioned sustained ethical debate (Kass 2004: 233–5), notably resource allocation (Faden and Kass 1991), epidemiology (Gordis et al. 1977), screening (Skrabanek 1988), health education (Doxiadis 1990) and health promotion (Williams 1984). Otherwise, ethical concerns about public health tended to arise in a rather piecemeal fashion, mainly when new public health challenges raised ethical questions about policies and practices. An example is the HIV/AIDs pandemic in the West in the 1980s, which generated worries about compulsory testing, mandatory reporting, and quarantining (Bayer et al. 1993; Levine and Bayer 1985; Faden and Kass 1991). But around 1990, there was increased recognition of, and concern about, the fact that the ethical dimension of public health had been underplayed when medical ethics segued into bioethics in the 1960s (Gillon 1990; Skrabanek 1990; Hall 1992; Horner 1992; Cole 1995). The upshot was the coalescence of ethical concerns about public health into a more concerted academic effort that eventually gave rise to the subfield of public health ethics.

Around 2000, there was another upsurge of interest as various professionals – notably, scholars and public health practitioners – started to clarify and analyse more closely the ethical aspects of public health (Kass 2001; Callahan and Jennings 2002; Childress et al. 2002; Roberts and Reich 2002). This is now manifested in the usual academic contexts. There is substantial research output in books (Chadwick and Levitt 1998; Beauchamp and Steinbock 1999; Bradley and Burls 2000; Gostin 2002a) and journals (for example, a journal, *Public Health Ethics*, is dedicated to the subject). Serious academic conferences are devoted, either exclusively or largely, to public health ethics. And the state of public health ethics curricula is a source of considerable and ongoing debate (Coughlin 1996a; Coughlin et al. 1997, 1999; Hyder 2000; Kessel 2003). This sharper focus on the ethics of public health has also informed Guidelines and Codes of Conduct for public health practitioners (Public Health Leadership Society 2002; Thomas et al. 2002). Consequently, the ethics of public health is a new and developing, but increasingly firmly established, feature on the landscape of medical ethics.

Consensuses

Although public health ethics is a nascent discipline there is consensus on two things. First, public health presents distinctive ethical challenges, not just moral problems already familiar from medical ethics and bioethics (Charlton 1993; Lachmann 1998; Lane et al. 2000; Holland 2010a). To explain, recall the point made above that public health is a distinctive branch of health care because it takes the population perspective. As a consequence of this, public health sometimes promises benefits, in terms of the health of target populations, at a cost to individuals. This creates dilemmas between the rights and needs of the individual and the rights and needs of the community. Of course, such dilemmas neither always nor necessarily arise because, happily, the rights and benefits of individuals and communities can coincide; so, public health is not intrinsically ethically dubious. Nor is public health unique in this regard, because dilemmas between individual and community arise in other contexts where public and private interests interface. Nonetheless, there is a consensus that the distinctive core of public health ethics is the trade-off that can arise between, on the one hand, protecting and promoting the health of populations, and, on the other, avoiding individual costs of various kinds, including physical danger, moral harm and frustrated desires (Schmidt 1995; Horner 1998, 2000).

The second consensus is related to the first. Because public health and, consequently, public health ethics are distinctive, it would be a mistake simply to apply the familiar findings of medical ethics and bioethics to public health problems (Thomas 2003). In particular, as mentioned above, advances in medical ethics and bioethics are due in large part to an increased awareness of, and concern to protect, individual rights grounded in ethical principles. For example, clinical medical research and practice have been modified in response to the recognition of an individual's right to consent, grounded in the principle of respect for autonomy. But, as just outlined, the distinctive thing about public health ethics is the dilemma that can arise *between* individual rights and community benefit. So, simply to apply the guiding principles of medical ethics and bioethics to the field of public health ethics would be to beg the question; i.e., it would be tantamount to assuming the priority of individual rights over communal benefit, when it is precisely the relative value of these that forms the core ethical question in the public health field. Consequently, pursuing public health ethics will require more imagination than applying templates borrowed from medical ethics and bioethics.

It is worth dwelling on this for a moment. There is a consensus on the fact that it would be question-begging to assume uncritically that the established principles of medical ethics and bioethics should guide public health ethics. However, when writers address quite how medical ethics and bioethics on the one hand, and public health ethics on the other, relate to one another, a range of views emerges. Some writers suggest that public health ethics is diametrically opposed to any other kind of health care ethics; others adopt a more conciliatory tone (Kass 2001; Levin and Fleischman 2002; Callahan and Jennings 2002; O'Neill

2002; Bayer and Fairchild 2004; Leeder 2004). It is sensible to take a balanced view here. On the one hand, the wholesale application of the principles and paradigms of medical ethics and bioethics to public health ethics – and no further type of analysis – would be inadequate. On the other hand, medical ethics and bioethics are not at loggerheads with public health ethics. For example, individual rights, which are so prominent in medical ethics and bioethics, are obviously important in public health too: the distinctive core of public health ethics – individual versus community – would not arise otherwise. So, some of the principles and paradigms of medical ethics and bioethics will be useful in analysing public health ethics problems, and public health ethicists should remain open to possible synergies here. Conversely, there has always been concern amongst some medical ethicists and bioethicists that individual rights in general, and the principle of autonomy in particular, have been allowed to overshadow more community-oriented goods and values. This concern is manifested in various ways, including criticisms of over-reliance on individual-oriented ethical principles (Callahan 1984; Gauthier 2000) and alternative 'schools' of bioethics, such as 'critical bioethics' (Parker 1995; Hedgecoe 2004). So, public health ethics, which naturally promotes communal values and a societal perspective, can reinvigorate and re-orientate bioethics; hence Wikler's (1997) depiction of 'a bioethics of population health'.

Justifying public health interventions

Public health ethics as understood in this book is taken to be about justifying public health interventions aimed at protecting and promoting population health in Western countries such as the UK and USA. As Horner (2000: 52) puts it: 'Every proposed new public health intervention should be carefully evaluated for its "ethical dimension".' Often, such interventions enjoy governmental support. Familiar contemporary examples include legislation banning smoking in public places, screening adults for obesity, testing would-be immigrants for HIV, funding epidemiologic research into genetic predisposition to late-onset disorders, and quarantining to contain the SARS outbreak. The central question is, ought we to go in for such-and-such a public health initiative? If so, on what grounds? If not, why not? How ought we to proceed when a public health policy promises community benefits but at a cost to individuals? What kind of analysis is appropriate to the question as to which of our public health practices are justified? So, in this book public health ethics is taken to centre on a justificatory exercise, i.e., the exercise of justifying our public health interventions.

This focus might seem too narrow. There are at least three worries to distinguish here. The first is about the focus on interventions, given that it is well known that health status is affected by much more than health services, no matter how public. The second worry is about the lack of focus on inequities and inequalities, given that public health's population perspective has encouraged a clear perception of the socio-cultural-economic determinants, such as class, race and poverty, of health status (Anand et al. 2004). And the third is about the focus on the First World when, if we are serious about pursuing public health, 'public' should include what Wikler describes as the '5 and ¾ billion human beings, all of whom we suppose are equal to us [but who are] unaccounted for and indeed unmentioned' (Wikler 1997: 186–7; cf. Leon and Walt 2001; Kass 2004: 237–9). Putting all this together, the way public health ethics is understood in this book might seem unsatisfyingly narrow: a proper ethics of public health would be conceptually, politically and geographically ambitious, and advocate global change for the sake of global health.

These important worries should not be disregarded. Perhaps nothing could be said to convince a highly politicized reader – what Wikler (1997) calls a reformer, as opposed to a scholar – of the putatively narrow focus of this book. But a case for the defence can be built. Nothing in the approach to public health ethics taken in this book is inimical to a more radical agenda of global reform. The overall aim, shared by everyone interested in public health, is to make the world a better place. A detailed ethical analysis of our public health interventions is one expression of that aim. Reducing inequities in the health of white and black Americans is another. Decreasing the prevalence of HIV in sub-Saharan Africa by empowering women is a third. And so on. These are clearly compatible projects. There is a second important point. It is easy to postulate a very stark choice: public health ethics is about the problems of either the First or the Third World. Underpinning this is the assumption that these two geo-political regions face very different challenges. Undeniably, there are major differences between First and Third World experience. But it is increasingly recognized that they are unavoidably interconnected in numerous ways (O'Neill 2002). Many so-called 'Third World' problems are prevalent in the First World, so the image of an 'us and them' that underpins an 'either–or' choice between global and Western public health is increasingly unrealistic. Given this, analysis and reforms relevant in the one domain are applicable in the other, and, to a substantial extent, to develop a discourse of public health ethics with 'our' problems in mind is, at the same time, to develop a globally applicable discourse.

So, what might at first blush seem a narrow approach to public health ethics can be defended. But there is one thing to retain from the critic's complaint. The radical agenda of reform the critic advocates can and should inform the ethical analysis of public health interventions that is our focus in this book. That agenda is based on a clear perception of health inequalities and the extent to which health is determined by oppressive political, economic, cultural, etc., structures and ideologies. So, one dimension of ethical analysis is the extent to which public health policies and practices help emancipate people from inequities and oppression. Take, for example, health communication campaigns that form part of a health promotion strategy (see Chapter 7). If it is the affluent, assertive middle classes who will pick up on the information and can better afford healthy food (which is more expensive), we can predict that the campaign will worsen health inequalities. This becomes an independent datum in our ethical analysis that counts against the programme (Guttman and Salmon 2004: 549–50). So, the radical agenda is firmly in place as part of the backdrop to the discussion.

Frameworks and human rights

The point was made earlier that, however open we are to synergies, we cannot simply import the established guiding principles of medical ethics and bioethics into the public health arena. Given this, how are we to pursue public health ethics? Two suggestions are firmly embedded in the literature. First, some writers advocate constructing a new ethical framework specific to public health. The idea is that, since the ethics of public health is distinctive, it requires a new analytic framework (Gostin and Lazzarini 1997). There are various worthy examples. Kass (2001) proposes a six-step framework, 'an analytic tool, designed to help public health professionals consider the ethics implications of proposed interventions, policy proposals, research initiatives, and programs'. So, concerning a public health programme, Kass recommends enquiring into its goals, effectiveness and burdens; looking at alternatives to the programme; and querying whether it is implemented fairly, and whether benefits and burdens associated with it are justly distributed. Another very clear suggestion comes from Childress et al. (2002: 171), who discern 'a loose set of general moral considerations – clusters of moral concepts and norms that are variously called values, principles, or rules – that are arguably relevant to public health'. Such considerations include producing benefits, distributing benefits and burdens fairly, and protecting privacy and confidentiality. Childress et al. discuss the applicability of such considerations; specifically, they propose five justificatory conditions 'to help determine whether promoting public health warrants overriding such values as individual liberty or justice': effectiveness, proportionality, necessity, least infringement, and public justification (p. 173).

Proposals for a framework for public health ethics such as these are laudable. They bring into focus the need to nurture a species of medical ethics appropriate to public health, and they contain good insights and suggestions. But 'framework' is a metaphor that implies an extant and rigid construction when, arguably, this is not altogether appropriate for a nascent and inchoate discipline such as public health ethics. Any framework may fit current and new ethical challenges in public health badly. Furthermore, talk of frameworks seems to get things the wrong way round: frameworks should emerge out of the developing practice of public health ethics, not vice versa. A better metaphor is suggested by Wikler: '[a bioethics of population health] may also require a new conceptual apparatus' (1997: 187). Wikler's point is that the conceptual apparatus familiar to bioethicists is not well suited to public health ethics, so bioethicists – or anyone else – undertaking public health ethics need to develop new ways of thinking and talking. This suggests linguistic metaphors, such as that public health ethics requires a new medical ethics discourse, better suited than talk of frameworks to the current state of public health ethics. There is nothing extant or rigid about the new language of public health ethics that medical ethicists and others will have to learn. The discourse of public health ethics will be shaped by the distinctive ethical challenges public health presents: useful concepts and ways of talking will develop whilst inappropriate, useless ones will fall away (cf. Martin 2004; Jennings 2003).

A second approach to ethical challenges in public health advocated by numerous influential writers employs the notion of human rights (Mann 1995; Gostin 2000, 2002a; cf. Gruskin and Loff 2002). Again, there is much to applaud about this. A rights-based approach to public health intervention is intended to achieve two things. First, it has the practical intent of protecting and promoting population health, the idea being that the most effective way to improve public health is by enforcing human – i.e., universal – rights to such things as health and health care. Second, it has the intent of basing population health on a sound moral basis, since rights are obviously ethical. Nonetheless, there are some problems with a rights-based approach to public health ethics. For one thing, '[h]uman rights do not have secure status in contemporary philosophical thinking about social justice' (Wikler 1997: 187). Furthermore, even if they did, rights often conflict with one another. But on the other hand, perhaps such problems are not very deep because all that is required here is to think harder about rights themselves, and how to trade them off against one another.

However, there are bigger worries about the rights-based approach. First, the main point in its favour is that rights seem tougher than ethics. For example, rights can be enshrined in law and backed by legal sanction. So, whereas ethics tends to be a rather rarefied subject lacking impact, rights can be practically efficacious. But this point in favour of the rights approach is vulnerable. The main agent for protecting rights is the State and, unfortunately, it is all too common for States to fail in this regard, either deliberately because human rights are inconvenient to them, or simply by being too weak. This still leaves open the possibility that an agent other than the State will fill the vacuum, but, as O'Neill (2002: 42) points out, this is depressingly unlikely. There is a second, conceptual difficulty. Rights are notoriously ambiguous. And the only way to disambiguate rights talk is to determine the obligations that a putative right enshrines. For example, the only way to interpret 'the right to health care' is to determine '*who* has to do *what* for *whom*' (O'Neill 2002: 42). But this implies that obligations, and not rights, are fundamental (cf. Leeder 2004: 437–8). O'Neill (2002: 42) sums up the point in a resounding phrase: 'Taking rights as basic to ethics, including health care ethics, does not get close enough to the action'. Third, there is a danger of merely restating the dilemma at the core of public health ethics, in terms of rights. As stated above, the dilemma is between individual and community. Suppose we assert human rights, for example to maximal health status. In pursuing that human right, we will be drawn to interventions that improve population health. The worry is that we can do so only at the cost of transgressing individual rights to privacy, liberty, confidentiality or whatever. Then the question will be, which is the important right, the human right to maximal health or the individual right to liberty? But this is just the core dilemma in public health ethics again, put in terms of rights.

At this point we need a light touch. It would be a mistake to think that we have to elect one or other approach to public health ethics, thereby eschewing the others. Talk of frameworks is helpful; perhaps a framework suited to ethical problems in public health will develop from work in this area. Talk of human rights is helpful and we should be alert to the role of rights in the developing discourse of public health ethics. So, better to be aware of, and remain open to, talk of frameworks and human rights, rather than thinking we have to adopt either, or some other, as our preferred approach.

The structure of this book

The overall aim of this book is to introduce and discuss theoretical perspectives on, and substantive issues within, public health ethics. To this end, the book is in two parts. Part I explains the moral and political philosophy most pertinent to public health ethics; the second part discusses the ethical dimension of the most important types of public health activities. It is worth making explicit some points about this structure. First, the general idea is that public health ethics must be informed by moral and political philosophy. This is not to relegate the role of case studies of specific public health interventions; after all, the ultimate point of public health ethics is to analyse the ethical aspects of actual and proposed public health activities. But, nonetheless, it is better to get some moral and political philosophy under our belts first because, otherwise, discussions tend to degenerate into a clash of intuitions and opinions about specific case studies.

A point about what is left out of this book is worth making. Although the book tries to be wide-ranging, it cannot be an exhaustive or comprehensive discussion of major public health topics. Specifically, some issues very pertinent to public health have been left aside because they are dealt with by neighbouring sub-disciplines. So, for example, resource allocation and rationing are not included here because these issues are so thoroughly discussed in health economics. Similarly, issues such as the gamete donor's putative right to anonymity are important public health matters, but not included here because they are debated by bioethicists. Generally, as this Introduction has tried to make clear, the urgent need is to develop a discourse of public health ethics; there is less urgency about the topics left out of this book because they are being worked on in cognate disciplines.

Part I Moral and
Political Philosophy

Introduction to Part I

The aim of Part I is to introduce, explain and discuss the moral and political philosophy most pertinent to public health ethics. It is important to have a clear overview of these first four chapters. First, we need to distinguish between moral philosophy, on the one hand, and political philosophy on the other. Chapters 1 and 2 deal with moral philosophy; Chapters 3 and 4 deal with political philosophy. Second, we need to be clear about how the material in Part I is organized. The discussion gets going with what will be called the naïve utilitarian view of public health. Utilitarianism is a consequentialist moral theory (such jargon is fully explained below) that says, roughly, the right thing to do is that which will maximize benefit. The naïve view is that any public health intervention is fully morally justified on the utilitarian grounds that it produces benefit by protecting and promoting the public's health. All the material discussed in Part I can be related back to this view. First, Chapter 1 criticizes this naïve utilitarian view of public health by discussing considerations from within the same moral philosophy framework to which it belongs, i.e., from within consequentialism. So, the rest of Chapter 1 explains more sophisticated versions of utilitarianism in order to query the naïve utilitarian view.

Chapter 2 is similar to Chapter 1 in that it, too, queries the naïve utilitarian view of public health. Also, it does so by appealing to theories in moral philosophy. But the important difference is that Chapter 2 moves beyond the consequentialist framework to which utilitarianism belongs by discussing *non*-consequentialist considerations that count against the naïve view. Specifically, three non-consequentialist moral theories which are very important to public health ethics, and which put pressure on the naïve utilitarian view, are explained and discussed. The first is called deontology (again, such unfamiliar jargon words are fully explained below). Deontology captures the idea that a public health intervention might be unethical just because of the kind of intervention it is, as opposed to anything to do with its consequences. Famously, Immanuel Kant developed a sophisticated deontological moral theory; Kant's theory is introduced in Chapter 2, where its application to public health ethics is illustrated.

The two other non-consequentialist moral theories discussed in Chapter 2 are called principlism and virtue ethics. Principlism is very well known in medical ethics because of an influential book by Beauchamp and Childress that has been updated and published numerous times, called *Principles of Biomedical Ethics*. Their original idea is that certain principles are particularly pertinent to biomedical ethics, so a proper discussion of ethical problems in biomedicine requires clarifying these principles and seeing how they apply in particular cases. Principlism has many strengths as an approach to biomedical ethics, but how well does it apply to public health? It is argued in Chapter 2 that Beauchamp and Childress's original biomedical principles are not well suited to public health; nonetheless, principlism is still important because other principles, better suited to public health ethics problems, can be developed. These other principles are explained and discussed, and their application illustrated.

Virtue ethics – the third non-consequentialist moral theory discussed in Chapter 2 – has a much longer history than principlism. In fact, virtue ethics is our oldest moral tradition, being rooted in ancient Greek thinkers such as Aristotle, and enjoying prominence in the neo-Aristotelianism of the Middle Ages. The basic idea behind virtue ethics is that morality is a matter of character; specifically, right action is that which is undertaken by the moral agent who acquires virtues, such as kindness and courage, and exercises them appropriately. This theory might seem too personal to be of much relevance to public health. But, on the contrary, some writers have argued that virtue ethics is the most important moral theory in public health ethics. And, as we shall see – for example, in the discussion of the ethics of epidemiologic research towards the end of Chapter 5 – virtue ethics is certainly pertinent to contemporary public health practice.

So, by the end of Chapter 2 we will have considered both conse-quentialist and non-consequentialist grounds for querying the naïve utilitarian view that all public health interventions are justified by protecting and promoting the public's health. Chapter 3 is in the same vein, but there are two important things to note here. First, as men-tioned above, Chapter 3 moves beyond moral philosophy and into political philosophy. Second, Chapter 3 starts with an argument called the liberal objection. The liberal objection is an objection to public health interventions based on the claim that they amount to an assault on individual liberties. So, as with the material in Chapters 1 and 2, here we have a response to naïve public health utilitarianism: liberty-limiting public health interventions are objectionable infringements on individual freedoms, whatever other good consequences they might have in terms of protecting and promoting the health of populations.

The question central to Chapters 3 and 4 is, how strong is the liberal objection to public health intervention? First, the political philosophy from which the liberal objection emanates, namely, liberalism, is defined. This is not such an onerous task because liberalism is the very familiar backdrop to our Western political culture and institutions. Then, grounds for questioning the strength of the liberal objection are considered. First, grounds for questioning the strength of the liberal objection found within liberalism itself are discussed in Chapter 3. One such is especially important in public health ethics, namely, Mill's harm principle. Bluntly, the harm principle says that the State is justi-fied in interfering in individual liberties to avoid harm to third parties. This has proved an enormously influential idea in Western political culture in general, and it is frequently appealed to in public health ethics (for example, it emerges numerous times in the discussions of important types of public health activity in Part II of this book). The principle is explained in Chapter 3, where its impact on the liberal objection is discussed. Another way of querying the liberal objection – again, still within the liberal tradition – focuses on how to understand the concept of freedom. The liberal objection rather assumes that freedom is merely the absence of constraints on individual choice. This is known as a negative conception of freedom because it defines freedom as the absence of something (i.e., constraint). But there are plausible positive conceptions of freedom, some of which are can-vassed in Chapter 3. The liberal objection looks much less compelling when freedom is defined positively.

Chapter 4 continues to apply political philosophy but here we move out of the traditional liberal circle of ideas to critique the liberal objection. First, we look at a recent and influential attempt to combine the liberal insistence on individual freedom with the paternalistic urge to get people to behave in their own best interests. This is 'libertarian paternalism' but it is also known by the less technical term, 'nudge'. Theoretical objections to, and applications of, 'nudging' are discussed. In the latter part of Chapter 4, liberalism is juxtaposed by a non-liberal political philosophy known as communitarianism. Communitarians criticize liberals for unreasonably emphasizing the individual and his or her freedom of choice. The general aim of the communitarian critique of liberal individualism is to re-establish the communal goods and values suppressed by liberalism's emphasis on individuals and their rights. Some of the details of this critique are explained, and its influence on public health policy evaluated.

1 Consequentialism

This chapter starts by explaining the theory in moral philosophy called consequentialism. Then a specific version of consequentialism, i.e., utilitarianism, is clarified. Given this, the naïve utilitarian view of public health can be presented. The naïve view is that policies and programmes that maximize public health gain are morally permissible, even morally obligatory. The rest of the chapter queries this naïve view by presenting constraints on the pursuit of maximal public health gain from within the consequentialist tradition to which it belongs. In other words, more sophisticated versions of utilitarianism rule out some public health activities, despite the health gains they can be expected to produce. Let's start with some definitions of basic terms.

Defining consequentialism and utilitarianism

Consequentialism is a major moral theory that states that the moral value of an action is determined solely by consequences (Rachels and Rachels 2007: 89–116). 'Action' is here used as an umbrella term for whatever it is the morality of which is in question, which can include single acts, motives, policies, regulations, laws and public health interventions. Examples of the 'moral value' of an act include being right, wrong, permissible, obligatory and supererogatory. This all sounds rather technical, but a virtue of consequentialism – an odd word, but actually quite a helpful piece of academic jargon – is that it captures a very natural and familiar line of thought. All of us have been faced with a moral situation in which we are puzzled as to the right thing to do; consequentialism says, in such circumstances, look only to the consequences of the available actions. The right thing to do is that which will bring about the best consequences. The wrong thing to do is that which will fail to bring about the best consequences.

Left at this, consequentialism is not much use because, unless we explain what makes a set of consequences good, or better than others, the idea that one ought to bring about the best one is unhelpful. This is where utilitarianism comes in. Utilitarianism is the example, or version, of consequentialism that states that what makes a set of consequences good is that it maximizes 'utility'. 'Utility' – a rather old-fashioned word – is often translated in terms of pleasure, happiness and, conversely, freedom from pain. But, since such terms make the theory sound hedonistic in a somewhat shallow sense, better phrases are well-being, welfare and benefit. So, utilitarianism is the version of consequentialism that says that the right action is that which brings about the best consequences, and the best consequences are those that maximize well-being, welfare or benefit.

Further clarifications

Before applying utilitarianism to public health, some further clarificatory remarks are called for in order to avoid misunderstandings. Firstly, utilitarianism is an impartial (or impersonal) theory. To explain, suppose someone were to ask whose welfare we are supposed to bother about, or whose well-being counts for most, when making a moral decision. The answer, according to utilitarianism, is that the well-being of everyone affected by the action in question counts and, moreover, counts equally. This is one of the most appealing aspects of utilitarianism: it is impartial (or impersonal) in the sense of denying that the welfare of some individual(s) or type(s) of people is more important than that of others. So, utilitarianism does not say that the right action is that which maximizes well-being for myself, or white people, or straight people or the able-bodied, or whomever; rather, it says that we should impartially maximize well-being.

To counter another possible misunderstanding, consider an imaginary scenario. A moral agent is walking quickly towards a class that is about to start. They see a frail, elderly person having difficulty crossing a busy road. The agent decides to stop, risking missing the start of their class in order to help. Halfway across, and without any warning, a drunken driver comes careering down the road, heading straight for them. The agent manages to dive out of the way but the elderly person is hit and injured. Did the agent do the morally right thing, according to utilitarianism? According to what might be called classical utilitarianism, the answer is, no, because utilitarianism says that the right action is that which maximizes benefit and, in this case, benefit was not maximized. But this might seem counter-intuitive. Here, it is useful to distinguish acting so as to maximize actual benefit and acting so as to maximize expected benefit, in order to suggest that we ought to act so as to maximize expected, not actual, utility. In helping the elderly person across the road the agent had every reason to expect to provide benefit (a safe passage) at a small cost (being late for class). So, according to this, arguably more intuitive, utilitarian account, the agent did the morally right thing, despite the actual, unfortunate outcome of their action.

Another point can cause confusion. Many people associate utilitarianism with the phrase, 'the greatest good for the greatest number'. To explain the misunderstanding that can arise here, consider another, rather more fanciful scenario. Imagine that a moral agent possesses the last 5 ml of a drug. What makes the drug unusual is that if 1 ml of it is given to each of five people, it has the effect of curing their common colds quite quickly, but if all 5 ml of the drug is given to one person who has a certain life-threatening condition, it has the effect of saving their life. Which should the agent do according to utilitarianism: give 1 ml to each of the five people, or all 5 ml to the one person? A natural line of thought is that, to do the greatest good for *the greatest number*, the agent should give 1 ml to each of the five people, because that way they help more people. But this is not correct. The utilitarian is interested in maximizing benefit *per se*, rather than maximizing the number of people who get some benefit from one's actions: i.e., it is about *the greatest good*, not the greatest number. So, because saving a person's life is of immeasurably greater benefit than getting over a cold a bit quicker, the utilitarian would conclude that the right action is to give all 5 ml to the one person.

The idea that the right thing to do is to maximize well-being is known as the principle of utility; and the weighing up of the expected utility of actions is called the utilitarian calculation. One might well complain that it is unrealistic of the utilitarian to expect us to do a utilitarian calculation every time we have to do something. Often, we simply do not have the time, energy or information to do so; and this might seem to imply that most of us are, for the most part, acting immorally. This is part of a general 'over-demandingness' objection to utilitarianism that we revisit in Chapter 9, in the context of a discussion about whether there is a general duty not to infect others. But, in the present context, suffice to say that the utilitarian can recognize the role of what are called 'rules of thumb' in moral deliberations. Take the example of turning up to work on time. Do we really need, every day, to calculate that being punctual maximizes expected utility? It is easy to notice that, generally speaking, being late for work causes problems to patients, colleagues and even ourselves that can be avoided simply by being on time. Given this, we should act according to the rule of thumb, I ought to get to work on time, rather than having to recalculate the same moral equation and getting the same result over and over again. The point to note is that this is still utilitarianism because what makes it right to act according to such a rule of thumb is that, in our experience, doing so tends to maximize well-being.

There are numerous objections to utilitarianism, debate about which is a massive industry in moral philosophy (see Rachels and Rachels 2007). There is not space to go deeply into this, which is not central to our concerns. But, to give a flavour of the discussion, recall the point made above about impartiality: utilitarianism aims at benefit, so it does not endorse preference for, or prejudice against, individuals or even types of people. This is said to be a virtue of the theory, but it is also a source of criticism. In one respect, this is another example of the general over-demandingness objection to utilitarianism, mentioned above. But the more pertinent objection here is that utilitarianism must be a false theory because it is at odds with some of our strongest moral intuitions. For example, people value their children's welfare much more highly than that of strangers, and it is not clear that to do so is to be immoral (this phenomenon is known as 'agent-relativity'). Utilitarians devise ways around the problem. One involves the notion of 'satisficing utilitarianism', which replaces the idea that the right action is that which maximizes benefit with the idea that an action is (all) right provided that it produces a satisfactory amount of benefit. This leaves open the possibility of being a utilitarian whilst preferring to benefit one's nearest and dearest: so long as the agent has acted so as to produce enough benefit given the circumstances, they can prioritize their loved ones even if they could have produced more overall utility by being wholly impartial. These are the kinds of debates in moral philosophy about utilitarianism; but rather than dwell on them further, let's apply utilitarianism to public health.

The naïve utilitarian view of public health

Public health, in spirit, principle and practice, is a utilitarian endeavour: 'Although public health measures have been undertaken for centuries, the philosophical basis of modern public health is generally considered to be nineteenth century utilitarianism' (Rothstein 2004: 176). The whole impetus behind public health is utilitarian – as Horner (2000: 49) puts it: 'Public health is basically utilitarian in character' – and, furthermore, '[f]or public-health professionals, this perspective has a strong intuitive appeal' (Roberts and Reich 2002: 1055). After all, the aim of public health is to benefit populations of people by protecting and promoting their health status. So, a simple formula suggests itself: utilitarianism says that the morally right thing to do is to maximize benefit; health is a benefit; therefore, any public health policy that will produce maximal health gain is morally justified (even obligatory). It seems that the problematic of this book – i.e., the justification for public health interventions – is not so problematic after all: a public health intervention is justified on the utilitarian grounds that it maximizes utility. Why not just leave it there?

Initial objections to the naïve view

Even if we stick with utilitarianism as introduced so far in this chapter, there is a very straightforward problem with this formula. One of the most basic objections to utilitarianism is that it is often very difficult to compare the utility values of dissimilar outcomes. Suppose, for example, £10,000 is given to a group of my students who are told to spend it so as to maximize utility. Various spending plans would be suggested: some want to go travelling, some want better academic resources, others want a very big party. All these plans produce similar amounts of benefit, but benefit of different, apparently incomparable kinds. How are we to decide which is the right thing to do with the money? Putting this in public health terms, utilitarianism has problems adjudicating between alternative public health policies that would create similar amounts of different kinds of health benefits.

This problem often arises because of scarce resources. Katz and Peberdy (1997: 93–4) have a nice example of a community health worker who only has resources sufficient for one of two projects, namely, setting up a playgroup or developing a service to counsel five individuals on their diet. According to utilitarianism, which should they do? They should maximize expected health benefit. But similar amounts of benefit would accrue from the two options. So, the question becomes, which is the most important or valuable kind of health benefit, the mental health of parents and the physical and emotional health of children to be gained from the playgroup, or the reduced risk of heart diseases and other illnesses due to the improved diet of the recipients of counselling? Utilitarianism, as presented so far, seems unable to answer this question.

That there are different kinds of incommensurable health benefits, and utilitarianism seems to lack the resources to adjudicate between them, is a problem that arises in, but is not restricted to, contexts in which resources are scarce. Charlton (2001: 59) has another good example (though he raises it for other purposes) which has nothing to do with resource scarcity. What is the right policy on the public availability of aspirin and paracetamol? The utilitarian answer is, whichever policy maximizes expected health benefits. But which health benefits are important? There are two main kinds, accruing to different sets of people. First, there is benefit in terms of pain relief to lots of people with minor conditions such as ordinary headaches. Second, there is benefit in terms of reduced incidence of paracetamol and aspirin overdosages amongst suicides. Which should we go for? Prioritizing pain relief implies a liberal public access policy; prioritizing suicide rates implies a conservative access policy. Let's assume that, in terms of benefit, the two options are fairly well balanced, so it is no use insisting that the right policy is that which maximizes benefit. In the end, we have to choose to prioritize one or other kind of health benefit, either explicitly as part of a discussion process, or as an implication of the policy we adopt.

Perhaps such trade-offs are not so difficult. After all, in such cases, whichever option is chosen, a good deal of utility in the form of health benefits has been created. If neither option is the winner in the sense of creating more health benefit, either is justified (recall the notion of 'satisficing utilitarianism' from the previous section). Also, these kinds of benefit trade-offs are diverting us towards theories of health rationing and prioritization, which are the domain of health economists. Let's change tack and look at some other considerations counting against naïve utilitarianism about public health. Recalling the simple formula mentioned a moment ago, the right thing to do is to maximize benefit; therefore, since health is a benefit, any public health policy that maximizes health gain is justified. This seems to suggest that even very Draconian public health measures are justifiable. For example, smoking is a public health problem, and there are enormous health benefits to be gained by eradicating smoking. So why not go the whole hog and ban cigarette production, outlaw smoking, refuse to treat smoking-related diseases, even publicly shoot a small number of smokers to deter the recalcitrant? Obviously, at least some of these policy initiatives are unethical. But why? Where do the constraints on the pursuit of utility in the form of maximal health benefits come from? As outlined in the Introduction to Part I, the key is to distinguish various kinds of constraints: the first kind stays within the consequentialist tradition, and we deal with those in the rest of this chapter; the next chapter looks at constraints on the pursuit of health from non-consequentialist ethical traditions.

Better consequentialist rejoinders to the naïve view

In the following discussion it will be useful to have a particular public health policy initiative in mind for purposes of illustration. Let's take the proposed policy of refusing to offer coronary artery bypass graft surgery to patients who refuse to promise to give up smoking (Underwood et al. 1993; Heath et al. 2002). Before going on to consequentialist considerations that count against this policy, let's expand a little on it. The principal motive for the policy is utilitarian. There are various ways in which the policy might succeed in producing maximum benefit. On the one hand, it might succeed in motivating the patient to quit. If so, the patient will avoid the adverse effects of smoking on their bypass graft, such as thrombotic occlusion, which would require an expensive, dangerous and relatively unpromising re-operation. On the other hand, if the recalcitrant patient is not treated, others stand to benefit. Notably, other patients stand to receive the scarce resources that would have been used up treating the smokers. So, let's say that it is at least arguable that utility is maximized by enforcing the policy. What consequentialist considerations count against it?

The first point to note is that, in the brief outline of naïve utilitarianism sketched so far in this chapter, we have said very little about the nature of consequences of actions. But when we reflect more on this, some salient points emerge. The first is that there is a tendency to think in terms of immediate or short-term consequences. But this is very unsophisticated. Consequences ramify; in fact, one of the most disconcerting features of moral life is that one's actions can initiate sequences of consequences that go far beyond the immediate. So it is with public policy. It might well be that refusing to treat smokers will achieve utility in the form of health gain in the short, and even medium, terms. But, arguably, the long-term consequences would be disastrous. For example, trust is a major factor in the success of any health system. One thing that grounds public trust in health systems is the belief that health professionals are committed to the treatment of conditions, not certain types of people. The policy in question chips away at these grounds for trust. It is not fanciful to suggest that the fabric of the health care system in which this public health intervention is implemented would unravel. Any short- or medium-term health gain achieved by the policy would be overshadowed by such a disastrous long-term consequence.

A second salient point to note is this. There is a tendency to restrict our view of consequences to those of a certain type. For example, in the present context, it is tempting to think only in terms of health-related consequences. But smoking has effects that are unrelated to health. Furthermore, many of these are beneficial (Charlton 2001). For example, smoking significantly enhances the social life of a very large number of people. It is understandable that health professionals are blinkered to this. But utilitarianism is not a theory explicitly about, let alone restricted to, health and medicine. What matters in utilitarianism is utility *per se*, not utility of a particular type. So, health benefits are very relevant, but only as relevant as other types or kinds of benefit. One way of putting this is, health is a good, but not the only good (i.e., we value things other than health). Nor is health necessarily the main good, the thing we value most highly (again, a truth to which health professionals are sometimes blinkered): 'Health is important as a component of well-being ... on any sensible view of [health and well-being] people trade off health against other goods' (Wilkinson 2009: 245). A consequentialist who values very highly something other than health would recommend policies that maximize benefit despite failing to produce maximal health gain. Recalling our case study, the point is that the health benefits of refusing to treat smoking-related diseases have to be put alongside the other costs and benefits of that policy, many of which are unrelated to health. It might be that the result of a utilitarian calculation restricted to health consequences is in favour of the policy, but a utilitarian calculation that includes all consequences – health-related and others – is not.

Rule-utilitarianism

So far, we have considered two consequentialist grounds for constraints on naïve utilitarianism about public health policies: when we build in long-term health-related consequences, and costs and benefits other than health-related ones, a more sophisticated utilitarian might eschew our illustrative policy of refusing to treat smokers. There is a third point that is somewhat more far-reaching, because it requires distinguishing between what are traditionally regarded as the two main versions of consequentialism, namely, act-utilitarianism (or direct utilitarianism) – which is the version we have been working with so far – and rule-utilitarianism. To explain, consider a thought experiment (McCloskey 1965; cf. Smart and Williams 1973). Imagine a deeply racist town divided between an affluent white community and their poor black neighbours. Relations between the two have degenerated into mutual hostility and suspicion. A truly heinous crime has been committed, say, the rape and murder of a white woman. The white community is outraged, convinced of the culpability of a particular black man. The town's sheriff has information that shows the suspect to be innocent, but which would not persuade the mob. If the sheriff were to publicly hang the man, the white community would be appeased. Otherwise, they will go on the rampage and commit terrible atrocities. According to utilitarianism, what ought the sheriff to do?

Utilitarianism seems to be in trouble here because the result of the utilitarian calculation is that the sheriff maximizes utility by hanging an innocent man; this is obviously immoral; so, utilitarianism must be a false theory. The utilitarian can appeal to the kinds of points already made in this chapter. For example, the point about long-term ramifications of one's actions can be invoked. No doubt the public hanging maximizes utility in the short, and even medium, terms. But what are the long-term consequences of this kind of expediency? What are the subtle effects on the integrity of the legislature? What would be the effects on this society if the expediency were discovered? Conversely, what long-term utility, in terms of setting an example of honesty and integrity, is lost by avoiding the high cost of a riot in the short and medium terms, and going ahead with the hanging? But such complications can be factored out. This is a thought experiment, so we can change the conditions to get at the salient points any way we like. So, let's stipulate that the expedient nature of the hanging is never discovered; the riot would be unspeakably awful, including multiple rapes and murders; the suspect, though innocent of this crime, was guilty of some other, and, if released, would go on to do terrible things, and so on.

Manipulating the thought experiment in such ways makes it untenable that utilitarianism, as understood so far, concords with our ethical intuitions. This is where rule-utilitarianism steps into the breach. The key to rule-utilitarianism is the distinction between acts and rules. As mentioned, 'acts' means individual actions, motives, policies, etc. But the rules invoked in rule-utilitarianism are those sanctioned because utility is maximized by society accepting and following them. So, according to the version of utilitarianism we have been dealing with so far, the focus is on the act (hence, 'act-utilitarianism') and the moral value of the action is evaluated directly in terms of its consequences (hence, 'direct utilitarianism'). But, according to the alternative version, i.e., rule-utilitarianism, the moral value of an act depends on whether it accords with rules. Two points are important here: first, this alternative is still a version of utilitarianism, because which societal rules are sanctioned depends solely on whether abiding by them maximizes benefit; and, second, this is 'indirect utilitarianism', in the sense that the act in question is not evaluated directly by reference to its consequences, but indirectly by asking whether it accords with the rules (Hooker et al. 2000).

The rule-utilitarian can deal with the thought experiment about hanging the innocent black man. The question for the rule-utilitarian is not about the direct consequences of that act itself. Rather, the question is, does the relevant action accord with rules sanctioned by society because they maximize utility? Clearly, the answer is no. Consider two candidates for part of the set of societal rules: punish according to guilt; punish according to expediency. Clearly, it is the former, and not the latter, which would form part of a set of rules sanctioned and followed because doing so maximizes utility. So, for the sheriff to hang the innocent black man would not be in accord with the relevant rules. Therefore, it is wrong on rule-utilitarian grounds.

Furthermore, it is easy to see how this shift from act- to rule-utilitarianism informs our deliberations about the illustrative policy of refusing to treat smoking-related diseases. Let's say, for the sake of argument, that the policy would accrue a significant amount of utility in terms of deterring smokers. We can even say that the direct consequences of refusing treatments would be maximum utility. Does this commit utilitarians to the rightness of the policy, and an obligation to pursue it? Not according to rule-utilitarianism. Consider two candidates for part of a set of rules for governing society's health services: first, when devising a treatment plan, take only a patient's condition into account; second, when devising a treatment plan, take into account what got the patient into that condition. The first, and not the second, would be sanctioned. And, crucially, this is so on utilitarian grounds: adopting and following a set of rules that included the former would maximize utility. So, a policy of refusing to treat smokers is ruled out by rule-utilitarianism. (For an application of rule-utilitarianism in a different public health ethics debate, see Parmet 2003: 1227.)

Concluding remarks

This chapter has introduced and clarified the moral theory at the heart of public health, namely, utilitarianism. The naïve utilitarian view of public health was presented. Three kinds of constraints on naïve utilitarianism about public health, all from within the consequentialist perspective, were delineated and illustrated. The first two constraints are discernible within act-utilitarianism; the third consisted of shifting from act- to rule-utilitarianism. We can extrapolate from this to a general strategy for analysing any public health intervention. Any viable public health policy or programme is proposed because it will produce utility in the form of public health. The three kinds of consequentialist questions raised in this chapter can be asked of it. First, what are the long-term ramifications of implementing that policy? Second, are there goods and values other than health that will be achieved by implementing or refusing to implement the policy in question? Third, even if the policy in question seems sound on act-utilitarian grounds, how does it look according to rule-utilitarianism?

2   Non-consequentialism

Consequentialist constraints of the kind outlined in the previous chapter are not the only resources within moral philosophy with which to resist the naïve utilitarian view of public health. Staying within moral philosophy, but moving outside consequentialism, there are plausible non-consequentialist moral theories that ground such resistance. This chapter introduces three non-consequentialist theories that can be adapted to inform public health ethics, namely, deontology, principlism and virtue ethics.

Deontology

Deontology appeals to a line of thought about ethics that is as natural and familiar as, but contrasts sharply with, consequentialism. The difference between these two moral theories lies in what they claim is the source of moral value. Consequentialism claims that moral value is determined solely by consequences; i.e., whether an action is right, wrong, obligatory, etc., is traced directly or indirectly to its consequences. By contrast, deontology claims that moral value can be independent of consequences. Specifically, the moral value of an action can depend on the nature of the action itself. Correspondingly, according to deontology, ethically speaking, some actions must be performed, and others must not, irrespective of any consequences. Given this, we can now make some sense of the strange word 'deontology', which is derived from an ancient Greek phrase that is usually translated as 'duty' or 'one must' (Rachels and Rachels 2007: 117–40; Langdridge 2000).

Deontology is appealing because it insists on a role for such obviously ethical notions as principles and duty. That some actions must be performed or avoided in principle, and that one must fulfil one's moral duty irrespective of the outcome, are ideas basic to both deontological ethics and ordinary moral thinking. There is a pitfall here. It is tempting to infer from this emphasis on principles and duties that deontology is the really *ethical* theory – the one that is really about morals – as opposed to a consequentialist theory such as utilitarianism which, by contrast, seems rather pragmatic and expedient. This is a mistake because both deontology and consequentialism are, equally, theories about ethics and morality, the difference between them lying in what they say makes an action morally right or wrong. According to deontology, an action can be ethical or unethical because of its very nature; by contrast, according to consequentialism, an action's moral value is never determined by the nature of the action itself, but by reference to consequences. There is a clear difference here, but not between a theory (deontology) that is about morality versus another (consequentialism) that is not.

It is worth pausing to illustrate this distinction between consequentialism and deontology. As is well known, Jehovah's Witnesses refuse to consent to blood transfusions. Imagine a clear-cut case in which a Jehovah's Witness is in dire need of a transfusion without which they will become very ill and die. How would a utilitarian approach the case? As the discussion in the previous chapter indicates, this is more complicated than might at first appear, because it depends on what version of utilitarianism is in play (recall the more sophisticated versions of act-utilitarianism, and rule-utilitarianism, from Chapter 1). Nonetheless, whatever version of the theory one subscribes to, according to consequentialism, the moral value of the various available actions traces back to consequences. But to the Jehovah's Witness patient, the blood transfusion is an action which, in itself and by its very nature, is ethically impermissible. Consequences are simply irrelevant to their moral evaluation. So, when the utilitarian health professional explains to the patient that the consequences of refusing the transfusion are that their painful, life-threatening condition will worsen, they get the deontological response that, nonetheless, religious principles and duty preclude consenting to the treatment.

A worry people often have about this illustration is that the Jehovah's Witness is in fact behaving like a consequentialist. On this account of the case, they are motivated to resist the blood transfusion because in so doing they increase the chances of their enjoying good consequences, such as getting to heaven, and avoid bad consequences, such as incurring God's displeasure. If this is the correct construal of the case, and the patient really is a consequentialist who is basing their action solely on its anticipated outcome, then it is not a useful illustration of deontology and should be abandoned for a better one. (Note, though, that it still would not be a case of utilitarian thinking: as explained above, utilitarianism is the impartial moral theory that an action is right in so far as it maximizes utility whereas, on this account, the patient is acting so as to ensure the best spiritual outcome for themselves.) But this consequentialist account does not seem like the right way to interpret the action. A devotee does not think in such a calculative manner but, rather, acts dutifully in accordance with religious proscriptions. This is why the patient would be offended by the thought that they refuse consent in order to curry favour with God or increase their chances of getting to heaven. For them, it is simply their duty to refuse the treatment because a blood transfusion is the sort of action which is, by its nature, wrong.

Kantianism

As was the case with consequentialism, deontology *per se* is not much use because there is little point in being told that moral value depends on the nature of the action in question until something is said about the kinds of actions that, by their very nature, are right or wrong. Again the example of the Jehovah's Witness patient is instructive. Most of us are not Jehovah's Witnesses. Of those of us who are not, some subscribe to different but equally strongly held religious convictions, whilst others are non-religious. So, to avoid letting deontological ethics degenerate into a series of stand-offs between people who ascribe moral value on the basis of the nature of actions differently, we need an account of what it is about an action that makes it intrinsically right or wrong that could apply to anyone. This is where Immanuel Kant comes in. Kant's moral theory is deontological because it is based on what he called 'the categorical imperative', i.e., the view that morality comprises a set of duties or obligations that are binding on us, categorically speaking, as opposed to requirements on us that are 'hypothetical' because they are binding on us only because they are means to an end. Furthermore, he based his account of morality on our faculty of reason rather than any particular set of convictions, such as religion; since we are all rational, Kant provides a way of developing the deontological approach to ethics that applies to all moral agents (Sullivan 1994).

How does Kant explain the moral value of actions? What kinds of actions are, by their very nature, right or wrong, according to Kant? For our purposes, two ideas are crucial. The first is that it is wrong to act in a way that treats others as mere means as opposed to ends-in-themselves. The second is that it is wrong to act in ways that cannot be universalized. So, now we have two ways of putting flesh on the bones of deontology: by its very nature, an action that treats others as means and not ends-in-themselves is morally wrong; by its very nature, an action that is non-universalizable is morally wrong. At first sight, these are odd ideas, so let's say a bit more about both before seeing how they can be applied in public health ethics.

Although we do not need to go into them in detail, Kant's grounds for ruling out actions that treat others as mere means are worth alluding to. Basically, Kant thought that people are made special by their distinctive capacity for personhood. 'Personhood' refers to a set of principally psychological capacities; although there is considerable debate about what these are, it is agreed that this set of capacities includes self-consciousness and rationality. Two things follow, on account of such capacities. First, persons are autonomous beings: i.e., they have the distinctive ability to think and act rationally, an ability best expressed, for Kant, when they behave morally or as member of the moral community. Second, they are valuable, in a distinctive way. Lots of things have exchange value; for example, the value of a coat is equivalent to the money someone would pay for it. But people have dignity, i.e., they are uniquely and intrinsically valuable, and have no exchange value. Even from this very brief overview, it is easy to see why Kant thought that to act in a way that treats someone as a mere means is, by its very nature, morally wrong: to do so undermines their autonomy and flouts their dignity.

The second idea that is useful to us was expressed by Kant as follows: 'Act only on the maxim through which you can at the same time will that it should become a universal law'. The key to unpacking this seemingly bizarre quote is to distinguish its three components: acts, maxims and universal laws. The act is whatever it is the morality of which is in question. Maxims can be thought of as principles or rules that one adopts to govern one's life. An important Kantian idea is that acts are not isolated, one-off events, but express, or are explained by, underlying maxims or principles. Which maxims is it our duty to act on? This brings us to the third component, universalizability. A basic requirement on, or test of, our duties is that the maxim in question could, in principle, become a universal law in the sense that it could be applied to, and be upheld by, everyone all the time. Kant explained that only some maxims are universalizable. This is because the universalization of some maxims involves one in self-contradiction. It is our duty not to act in ways that express non-universalizable maxims.

Here there is a complication. Kant distinguishes two ways in which an act might fail the universalizability test, which correspond to two kinds of self-contradiction. Kant called the first, contradiction in conception. To illustrate, consider an example Kant himself used. Suppose I govern my life according to the maxim, promise falsely for personal gain. This could be very useful to me; for example, I could borrow money having falsely promised to repay it. But what happens when I try to universalize the maxim? The result is the dictum: everyone always promises falsely. Is this possible? The problem is easy to see. What would happen to the practice or institution of promising if everyone always promised falsely? It would disintegrate. The only way I can successfully promise falsely is if there is an institution of promising, and that requires that people in general maintain the institution by promising sincerely. Once my dubious maxim is universalized, I am involved in self-contradiction: I aim to do something (promise falsely) that is impossible because there is no longer the required practice or institution (of promising).

Kant called the second kind of self-contradiction, contradiction in the will. To illustrate this, Kant mentions the maxim, look after one's own interests and refuse to help others in need of our assistance. Suppose, for example, I see some new neighbours moving in, struggling with lots of heavy boxes. I could help them or I could not. Acting on the maxim Kant mentions, I ignore them. The universalization of the maxim is, everyone always looks after one's own interests and refuses to help others in need of one's assistance. There is no self-contradiction of the kind that arose in the case of promising falsely. Specifically, there is no formal contradiction implied by universalizing the maxim, since it is logically possible for everyone to be unhelpful to one another. But there is still self-contradiction because, given the kind of creature I am, circumstances are bound to arise in which I want people's assistance. But when that occurs, in ignoring my new neighbours and thereby endorsing the universalizability of the maxim, I am contradicting myself. My action implies both that I do want the maxim to be universalized, and that I do not want it to be universally applicable (i.e., when I am the one in need of assistance).

There is an important point to note at this point about Kant's approach to ethics. People often think that what Kant had in mind is a sort of science fiction story in which everyone starts behaving in the same way. This interpretation takes the notion of universalizability too literally, as though the behaviour in question is liable to catch on with friends, family, neighbours, etc., until everyone is always acting in that way. But this is not Kant's idea. His is not a practical point about bad behaviour 'catching on'. Rather, the test of universalizability is a thought experiment that takes place in the mind as one ponders whether it is in principle possible to will that everyone always behaves according to one's maxims, the point being that self-contradictions arise in the process of thinking through the ramifications of universalizing one's principles.

There is another possible confusion about the two ideas – that we should never treat people as mere means, nor act on maxims that fail the test of universalizability – presented here. One might think that both ideas can be put in consequentialist terms. For example, one might rewrite them as follows: an act that has the consequence of treating people as means or as resulting in self-contradiction is morally wrong. But this is a mistake. It is true that there is a sort of consequence to treating others as means and acting on non-universalizable maxims, but on reflection it is easy to see that this is not the kind of consequence relevant to utilitarianism. Utilitarianism is concerned with the effect of actions in terms of well-being or benefit. By contrast, what makes actions right or wrong according to Kant is whether they flout the autonomy and dignity of others and whether they are based on universalizable maxims, and this moral value is impervious to whatever else might count in its favour, including beneficial consequences.

Kantianism and public health ethics

Both aspects of Kant's ethics described in the previous subsection can be adapted to apply in public health. Consider, first, the proscription on treating people as mere means. To an extent, this captures the very essence of public health ethics. As explained in the Introduction, the central dilemma in public health ethics is between individuals and populations. Very often, ethical concerns about public health arise because initiatives and policies are proposed and implemented that can be expected to maintain or improve the health of a target population, but at the expense of some of its individual members. In Kantian terms, such individuals are being used as means to an end – namely, population health – as opposed to ends-in-themselves. Recognizing the moral danger in public health of becoming insouciant about the fate of individuals, because of an overriding concern to achieve such ends as lower incidence and prevalence rates, is an important corrective to a naïve utilitarian approach:

> Utilitarianism ... simply justifies us in giving supremacy to the needs of the community in the belief that this will benefit most individuals. The minority of individuals who do not benefit, and who may indeed be harmed, also deserve our consideration. Ultimately, the utilitarian is obliged to argue, if a small number suffer so that the population group can prosper and flourish, then so be it. (Horner 2000: 50)

For example, suppose, there is a public health effort aimed at reducing the incidence of a disease by implementing a screening programme. The utilitarian instinct is to focus on the bigger picture – what Pellegrino (1995) calls 'the statistical morality of utilitarian politics' – by looking at such things as the current, projected and future incidence rates, with and without the screening programme. Implementing a policy of making screening compulsory might well maximize population health gain. But what about the individual who would not consent to be screened, perhaps because the anxiety it would induce outweighs putative benefits? There is a danger of treating that individual as a means to an end. The end is lower rates of incidence of the disease; the means is coercing them onto a screening programme. According to the Kantian doctrine, never treat others as means but always as ends-in-themselves, this is morally dubious. So, Kant's deontology helps shift focus from the utilitarian agenda of maximal health gain to proper respect for the individual: 'simple and unqualified consequentialist reasoning ... fails to take seriously the separateness and inviolability of persons' (Buchanan et al. 2000: 11).

How does the second of Kant's ideas, about universalizability, apply to public health ethics? Here it is important to distinguish two agents in public health: first, those who devise and implement public health programmes (such as health planners and government health agencies); second, individual members of target populations whose actions affect the health of their community. The test of universalizability applies to both, but somewhat differently. To illustrate the former, consider a straightforward application of the universalizability test to the illustrative policy from the previous chapter, i.e., the policy of refusing to treat certain smokers. The maxim this is based on is, provide treatment according to desert rather than health need. Is this a universalizable maxim? Arguably, assuming that we are dealing with

a needs-based health care system, it involves a contradiction in conception. The only way we can have a needs-based health care system is if
it is not the case that we always treat according to desert. To refuse to
treat smokers in the way suggested requires that, for the most part,
patients are being treated according to medical need – thereby maintaining a needs-based health care system – whilst making an exception
of this particular class of patients. This helps account for a familiar
reaction to this policy, namely, that it is discriminatory in selecting one
set of patients on the basis of their behaviours and refusing to treat
them, when other sets of patients behaving in equally dangerous ways
(people who play contact sports, for example) get the treatment
demanded by their conditions (cf. Epstein 1997; Cappelen and Norheim
2005). Arguably, there is a contradiction in the will here, too. When
the advocate of the policy falls ill, they want their health care to be
needs-based rather than dependent on how they behaved prior to
becoming ill. But in advocating the policy they will its universalization;
so, they are involved in self-contradiction.

Admittedly, this application of Kant's deontology to the case study
is somewhat awkward. The reason for this introduces a major objection to Kant's approach: it all rather depends on which maxim an act
is said to express. In the foregoing, it is assumed that the policy
expresses the maxim, base treatment on desert rather than health
need; it was shown that this generates contradictions when willed to
be universal law. But there are other ways of describing the maxim
expressed by the policy in question. Perhaps the relevant maxim is,
help sufferers break self-harming habits, or, ensure the most effective
allocation of scarce health resources. Willing the universalization of
these maxims does not seem to involve contradiction. This problem
– that the same action can be said to express quite different maxims
and this is crucial to the moral evaluation of the action, since it is the
maxim that is tested for universalizability – is quite general and not
just a feature of this particular illustration. Nonetheless, the fact that
more needs to be said about this application does not render the test
of universalizability irrelevant to the ethics of public health policy.
The general point is that Kantianism require us to look beyond the
policy in question to the maxims (i.e., principles) on which it is based,
to enquire into whether those maxims can be endorsed without
self-contradiction.

The other perspective just distinguished is that of individual members
of target populations whose actions affect the health of their community. The doctrine that it is wrong to act on maxims that cannot be
universalized without contradiction applies very well to public health

ethics cases – some of which are discussed more fully later in this book – that involve individuals 'free-riding'; i.e., where individuals enjoy the health benefits of communal undertakings without making the necessary contributions or incurring the necessary risks. A clear example is what Dare (1998) calls 'voluntary non-immunizers' who choose to opt out of mass immunization programmes, thereby enjoying the benefits of herd immunity without taking risks associated with the vaccine and incurred by 'voluntary immunizers'. As we shall see in Chapter 9, Dare suggests that the actions of a small number of voluntary non-immunizers are morally permissible. But this seems to assume consequentialism, whereas what accounts for our sense that such free-riding is morally dubious in itself is its non-universalizability: it is not the case that everyone can free-ride (if they did, there would be nothing to free-ride on). If this is right, and 'voluntary non-immunization' is immoral on Kantian grounds, there is support from deontological moral theory for coercive immunization policies.

The main point of this subsection is that deontology can be adapted to inform public health policy and practice. The hallmark of deontology is the thought that actions can be right and wrong by their very nature, and not only because of their consequences. Kant explains two types of actions that are wrong in themselves: actions that treat people as mere means, and actions that are based on non-universalizable maxims. Both can be adapted to apply to public health ethics cases. So, now we have a further, non-consequentialist theoretical perspective on public health ethics.

Principlism

As with deontological theories, principlism can be adapted to provide constraints on naïve utilitarianism in public health. First, we need to get the basic idea behind principlism, which is a well-established and influential approach to medical ethics (Beauchamp and Childress 2013; T.L. Beauchamp 1995; Gillon 1998). Beauchamp and Childress suggested that medical ethics problems can be approached by adhering to principles of biomedical ethics. They had no intention of over-simplifying matters by reducing complex dilemmas in health and medicine to a few principles. Rather, the idea is that there are certain principles that best reflect the important values at stake in such dilemmas, and that are most useful in resolving them. Beauchamp and Childress outlined four main principles, namely, the principles of respect for autonomy, beneficence, non-maleficence and justice (for further details on the four principles, see Singleton and McLaren 1995: 29–55; Macklin 2003; DeMarco 2005).

The inapplicability of the four principles of biomedical ethics

It is questionable as to how useful these four principles of biomedical ethics are in public health (cf. Coughlin et al. 1997: 3–7; Katz and Peberdy 1997: 89–101; Holt et al. 2000). Consider, first, autonomy. This is an important, but much disputed, philosophical concept that is influential in applied ethics in general and medical ethics in particular. Beauchamp and Childress (2013: 101) recognize that the precise meaning of 'autonomy' is undecided but say: 'At a minimum, personal autonomy encompasses self-rule that is free from both controlling interference by others and limitations that prevent meaningful choice, such as inadequate understanding.' So, the basic idea is that of self-rule ('autonomy' being Ancient Greek for 'self' + 'rule'), i.e., people's ability to step back from their situation and decide for themselves how to behave. But this basic idea can be, and has been, interpreted in quite diverse ways. In fact, we have already encountered this: as mentioned in the previous section, the Kantian proscription against treating others as mere means is grounded in their dignity as persons, which, in turn, is grounded in their autonomy. Although Kant's notion of autonomy is not quite that which figures in biomedical ethics, it shares the same roots. These, and all other interpretations of autonomy, express the basic idea that people should be respected for their ability to decide for themselves.

Happily, we do not need to go further into the analysis of the concept of autonomy here because it is fairly clear that the principle of autonomy is not going to be much use in public health ethics. Invoking the principle amounts to respecting and preserving people's ability to decide for themselves; conversely, we flout the principle when we unnecessarily restrict someone's ability to be self-determined. For example, in clinical ethics this is taken to ground the right to consent to treatment: to treat a competent patient without their voluntary and informed consent is to fail to respect their ability to decide for themselves what happens in and to their bodies. But, as outlined in the Introduction, the central ethical dilemma in public health arises precisely when we feel compelled to restrict individuals' autonomy in the interests of the community. So, invoking the principle of autonomy amounts to simply opting for the individual against the community, which is clearly no way to resolve the dilemma: 'This relentless drive towards autonomy takes us to the other end of our dilemma, from that of utilitarianism and, as such, does not resolve it' (Horner 2000: 50).

The next two of Beauchamp and Childress's four biomedical principles are the principles of non-maleficence and beneficence. The former 'obligates us to abstain from causing harm to others' (2013: 150). By contrast, the latter refers to 'a moral obligation to act for the benefit of others' (p. 203). So, roughly speaking, 'maleficence' means, do no harm, and 'beneficence' means, help others. There are a couple of points worth noting in passing about these principles. First, in health care contexts, harms and benefits involve more than just being in good health and free from ill-health, because people have other important interests, too, such as preserving dignity and being treated with respect. Second, and as Beauchamp and Childress are at pains to stress, 'non-maleficence' might seem a lot like beneficence, but it is subtly and importantly different: beneficence is about helping people whereas non-maleficence is about not harming them; and, often, the principle of non-maleficence is more stringent than that of beneficence because it is more important not to harm someone than it is to help them.

Once again, the details need not detain us because neither principle is very useful in public health ethics. We can see this by once more recalling the dilemma at the heart of public health ethics, between individual rights and communal benefit. Different 'important or legitimate interests' clash in such dilemmas: i.e., the interest the individual has in asserting their individual liberties clashes with an interest in the well-being of the community. Which should prevail? The principle of beneficence does not address this, so cannot help to resolve public health ethics problems. Likewise, to which 'evil or harm' should we attend: the harm of transgressing individual rights to decide to participate in public health endeavours, or the communal right to expect individuals to care for their communities? Again, the principle of non-maleficence cannot resolve this, so its use in public health ethics is very limited.

The story is the same for the fourth principle, the principle of justice. Beauchamp and Childress base the principle of justice on 'fair, equitable, and appropriate treatment in light of what is due or owed persons' (2013: 250). Justice, in this sense, is about people getting what they deserve. People can deserve all kinds of things (reward, punishment, treatment, compensation, information, etc.) for all kinds of reasons (they have earned it, they are owed a duty of care, they are your friend, etc.). We abide by the principle of justice by giving someone what they are owed, and flout the principle by failing to do so. But, once again, we have here a principle of biomedical ethics poorly suited to resolving the central dilemma in public health ethics. To see this, one only has to notice how the rhetoric of 'justice' is used both to protect individual liberties and to motivate community spiritedness. What do we owe people when individual rights and communal benefits collide? Is justice best served by allowing individuals their freedoms, or by imposing on individuals for the sake of the population as a whole?

Since the best-known biomedical principles turn out to be unsuited to public health ethics and, furthermore, principlism has been strongly criticized even as an approach to clinical ethics, we might simply abandon it. But this would be a shame because principlism has some important benefits. For one thing, it is well suited to alerting non-philosophical professionals to the ethical dimension of their specialty, a very pertinent point in the present context because ethics is currently underdeveloped in public health. Furthermore, principlism is a very practical approach because its heuristic nature makes application to real-world problems relatively straightforward. Given this, it would be better to adapt principlism by developing principles better suited to public health.

Principlism adapted

Upshur (2002) agrees that 'the straightforward application of the principles of autonomy, beneficence, non-mal[evolence] and justice in public health practice is problematic' (p. 101). Nonetheless, he retains principlism's general approach by describing four principles which, though by no means exhaustive of the ethical dimension of public health, 'seek to bring clarity to some of the ethical aspects of public health decision making in practice' (p. 102). Upshur's first principle is Mill's famous harm principle, which presents a general condition on restrictions by government (or governmental agencies) on the liberty of an individual or group: 'the only purpose for which power can be rightfully exercised over any member of a civilized community, against his will, is to prevent harm to others. His own good, either physical or moral, is not a sufficient warrant' (Mill 1975: 15). Mill's harm (or liberty) principle is so important in public health ethics that it is a major focus of the next chapter, so it will be better to postpone discussion of it until then.

Upshur's second principle is the principle of least restrictive or coercive means. The basic idea here is of a list of ways of intervening to achieve public health goals which goes in order of ethical preference from less to more coercive styles of intervention. Upshur illustrates this: 'Education, facilitation, and discussion should precede interdiction, regulation or incarceration' (p. 102). This condition on ethical public health intervention re-emerges in other literature on public health ethics. For example, part of the framework for public health ethics recommended by Childress et al. (2002) includes five justificatory conditions 'to help determine whether promoting public health warrants overriding such values as individual liberty or justice', one of which is 'least infringement[:] For instance, when a policy infringes autonomy, public health agents should seek the least restrictive alternative' (p. 173; cf. Childress and Bernheim 2003: 1202–6). And the same idea is presented as the 'intervention ladder' by the Nuffield Council (Nuffield Council on Bioethics 2007: 41–3). However, an oddity about Upshur's presentation is worth mentioning in passing. He claims: 'The principles articulated will not, for example, cover ... health promotion programmes.' But, as we shall see in Chapter 7, the principle of least restrictive or coercive means seems eminently well suited to a discussion of the permissibility of ways of attempting health behaviour modification.

Upshur's third and fourth principles are the reciprocity and transparency principles. The reciprocity principle states that 'society must be prepared to facilitate individuals and communities in their efforts to discharge their duties' (p. 102). The basic idea here is that compliance with public health requirements can be burdensome for individuals. The principle states that, where this is so, there are obligations on public health bodies (such as a public health department). For one thing, the public health institution should provide the means to enable individuals to comply, such as relevant information. For another, there may be an obligation on public health bodies to compensate individuals for the cost of their compliance with public health measures. Upshur's fourth principle, the transparency principle, puts various conditions on the process by which public health decisions are made: all stakeholders should be involved; all should have equal input into deliberations; decision making should be clear and transparent; decision making should be as free as possible from political and nonpolitical vested interest.

Other principles

The policy of retaining principlism without foisting Beauchamp and Childress's famous principles on public health has been recommended by other commentators, some of whom have suggested principles of public health ethics different from Upshur's (Schramm and Kottow 2001; Klugman 2002). One sensible approach taken in the literature is to borrow and adapt principles from outside the health field that seem well suited to public health. An example is the precautionary principle (PP), which is a response to developments in our dealings with the environment. Pressure to develop proper assessments of risks to the environment from human activities was created when a permissive attitude – i.e., that the environment is sufficiently robust to accommodate whatever humans do to it – gave way to increased awareness of serious environmental problems due to human activity. But, it transpired, science is unable to provide accurate environmental risk assessments. This is due to two kinds of scientific limitations. First, there are limits to current scientific knowledge; for example, requisite detailed, long-term research is lacking. Second, there are in-principle limits on scientific knowledge; for example, many natural processes are simply too chaotic to be fully understood and predicted. So, inevitably, human activities are undertaken under conditions of uncertainty about their environmental impact (J. Parker 1998; Mepham 2005: 317–23).

The PP – which developed as a response to this predicament – is elusive because it 'is wide ranging with many different interpretations and formulations' (J. Parker 1998: 633). Nonetheless, a good place to start is the prominent definition provided by the UN Conference on the Environment and Development in Rio de Janeiro in 1992, at which the principles comprising the Rio Declaration were formulated. Principle 15 is:

> In order to protect the environment, the precautionary approach shall be widely applied by States according to their capabilities. Where there are threats of serious or irreversible damage, lack of full scientific certainty shall not be used as a reason for postponing cost-effective measures to prevent environmental degradation.

The Rio Declaration captures a crucial element in the PP, namely, that since scientific uncertainty is inevitable, it should not be a consideration against preventive measures. But this interpretation of the PP is fairly weak; other formulations, by contrast, commit concerned parties to regulatory action. A case in point is the 1987 London Declaration on the Protection of the North Sea, which states that substances will be regulated 'where there is reason to assume that certain damage or harmful effects on the living resources of the sea are likely to be caused by such substances, even where there is no scientific evidence to prove a causal link between emission and effects'.

The PP emerges as 'a prototypical ethical principle' (J. Parker 1998: 634) motivated by reflection on environmental science, influential because widely accepted and appealed to in both politics and law, but as yet vague and capable of sustaining stronger and weaker versions depending on the speaker's ideology (Royal Society of Canada 2001; cf. Applegate 2000; Weed 2002/2003). It is also a principle that has received much academic attention (O'Riordan and Cameron 1994; Appell 2001; O'Riordan et al. 2001), including strong criticism (Guldberg 2000; Morris 2000). Nonetheless, Bayer and Fairchild (2004) suggest that the PP applies in public health:

> the [precautionary] principle has only recently been explicitly invoked in the context of epidemic threats where pre-emptive actions may burden individuals and impose limits on their freedoms. Nevertheless, the precautionary principle has implicitly guided public health interventions designed to limit or forestall epidemic outbreak. (P. 490)

According to Bayer and Fairchild, at least as far as the public health response to epidemics is concerned, the PP has always had an implicit role, and now has an explicit one. The example of the latter they cite is the 2002 SARS outbreak, when '[h]ealth officials had to act without full scientific knowledge about the nature of disease transmission' (p. 490). Officials invoked the PP: despite the inevitable uncertainty about SARS due to scientific limitations, they protected some populations by stringent measures, including isolation and quarantine (pp. 482–5).

Bayer and Fairchild's comments indicate a general application of the PP in public health (cf. Wynia 2005a). As we shall see in Chapter 5, the scientific uncertainty under which health officials responding to SARS laboured is typical in public health because of the epistemological difficulties in epidemiology. So, the basic motivation behind the PP – uncertainty due to scientific limitations – is in place in public health, just as it is in the biosciences. But interestingly, the typical effect of the PP in public health is exactly opposite to that in dealings with the environment. Generally, though not always, the point of invoking the PP in environmental science is to advocate caution, which often leads to inaction: i.e., lack of scientific certainty about the harmful effects of such-and-such is no reason to go ahead with such-and-such. By contrast, the point of invoking the PP in public health is to advocate caution leading to action: for example, lack of scientific certainty about the harmful effects of a disease is no reason not to go ahead with preventive public health interventions. Hence, the objections to invoking the PP in dealings with the environment are often the exact converse of objections to invoking the PP in public health. The biggest criticism of the PP is that it stymies scientific and technological progress by advocating caution under conditions of uncertainty. By contrast, a major problem with the PP in public health is that it permits overly intrusive, Draconian interventions. As Bayer and Fairchild put it: 'The challenge to the precautionary principle is illustrated by quarantine in the case of SARS. To avoid catastrophe, [health officials] took action that proved unnecessarily extensive' (2004: 490).

The PP is an example of how principlism can be retained despite the inapplicability of the traditional principles of clinical ethics to public health. Of course, this leaves much work to be done. Principles have to be defined and defended. And, even when there is a fairly straightforward application of one principle, there is always more to say because other principles can be invoked either to support or question the conclusion. This is alluded to by Bayer and Fairchild who, after their mention of the unnecessarily extensive action taken in response to SARS, comment: 'The only safeguard against the misuse of authority [in the name of precaution] is transparency and open acknowledgement that new evidence may necessitate a reconsideration of policies.' This recalls Upshur's fourth principle, the transparency principle, and illustrates the general point that principlism proceeds by way of an iterative dialogue between principles relevant to public health dilemmas.

Virtue ethics

Kantianism and principlism provide two non-consequentialist perspectives on public health ethics. Virtue ethics offers a third. Virtue ethics represents a perfectly natural and familiar line of thought. To feel our way into it, consider bringing up a child. One of the responsible parent's many concerns is to ensure that their child turns out to be a good person. What does this aspect of parenting entail? It seems to have relatively little to do with utilitarianism, deontology or principlism. True, parents sometimes point out the good and bad consequences of their child's actions in order to encourage or discourage certain types of behaviour. Likewise, parents sometimes say things like, 'that was selfish – what if everyone behaved like that?' But, for the most part, parents are getting their child to develop a certain kind of character, or to become a certain kind of person, by ensuring that they acquire virtues, i.e., character traits such as kindness, courage, honesty, and the like (a useful platitude here is, 'patience is a virtue').

Applying virtue ethics to public health

It is natural to think that virtue ethics is ill-suited to public health because it is a theory about personal morality. But, on the contrary, one influential commentator argues: 'Of [a number of schools of ethics] only virtue ethics, perhaps supported by the insights of feminism and the ethics of care, appear to help with [the central ethical dilemma in public health between individuals and community]' (Horner 2000: 48). Why does Horner think this? One negative factor is that he sees clearly that some ethical theories tend simply to endorse the claims of either the individual or the community, as opposed to genuinely resolving the dilemmas that can arise between these two claimants. We have already encountered this point: for example, one of the worries about applying utilitarianism in public health is that it 'simply justifies us in giving supremacy to the needs of the community' (Horner 2000: 50). So, what we need are not ethical theories that deny the dilemma by promoting one of its parts at the expense of the other; rather, we need ethical theories that allow a rich sense of how real the dilemma is in public health between individuals and communities.

In response, some specific features recommend virtue-based theories to Horner. First, virtue ethics is rooted in classical thought, and ancient Greek philosophers such as Aristotle argued for what is known as the Doctrine of the Mean. Roughly, this means that the virtuous agent is characterized as adopting the mean between two opposing vices. For example, one might be in a situation in which one could act in either of the following two ways. First, one might be courageous to the point of foolhardiness, rushing in and doing more harm than good. Second, one might lack courage to the point of cowardice, failing to do anything in a situation that demands action. Foolhardiness and cowardice are two opposing vices. The virtuous agent recognizes both extremes, but acts in a 'practically wise' manner by adopting the mean between the two. As Horner puts it, this 'should be the key to what we are seeking [in public health ethics] – a balance between two equally unsatisfactory extremes' (p. 50). The 'two equally unsatisfactory extremes' are advancing communal benefit without caring about the fate of individuals, and protecting individual rights without caring about communal benefits. The Doctrine of the Mean in public health involves sensitively balancing the claims of individuals and the claims of communities rather than rushing to adopt policies that can meet only one at the expense of the other.

A second feature that recommends virtue-based theories to Horner is referred to technically as non-codifiability. To illustrate, take an uncontentious virtue, that of being polite. How does a parent get their child to be polite? They neither do nor could present their child with a handbook that includes a list of situations in which, for example, it would be appropriate to say, 'thank you'. Rather, the parent gets the child to understand what it is to be polite by getting them to 'cotton on' to the very idea of politeness in such a way that the child can then go off into the world and be sensitive to those situations in which saying 'thank you' is appropriate. The story is the same for more interesting virtues, such as kindness. A parent neither does nor could write a handbook that describes all those situations that demand kindness, and what sort of kindly response would be appropriate. Rather, the parent's job is to get the child to latch on to the very idea of being kind in such as way that they recognize for themselves when kindness is required and what sort of response would be a kind one. In this way, the parent is moulding the child's character. Non-codifiability is one of the features that make Horner think virtue theories are best suited to public health:

> in seeking solutions to our dilemma [in public health between individuals and communities], we shall seek to pursue virtue. Sometimes this will allow us to give greater emphasis to community needs, whereas at other times we may emphasize the needs of individuals. (P. 50)

Horner's point is a good one. Of the major ethical theories on offer, virtue ethics scores well by not simply denying the central ethical dilemma in public health between individuals and communities, by recommending moderation between the more extreme pro-individual and pro-community positions, and by endorsing the flexibility required to respond sensitively to discrete public health dilemmas. He goes on to outline a sketch of the virtuous public health physicians who are 'fully aware of this conflict between the needs of the individual and those of the community and constantly try to address it' and 'seek to be truthful', and who 'demonstrate the virtue of courage, by constantly challenging both managerial and medical orthodoxy' (pp. 51–2). Here we see another advantage of Horner's endorsement of virtue ethics. Responsibility for responding to the central dilemma in public health ethics is placed firmly within the public health field – for Horner, it is the public health physician whose virtue is at stake – rather than with others, such as government agencies and chattering academics. After all, in the end, dilemmas in public health arise for public health professionals, and their responses are the ones that have the practical impact.

Generally speaking, virtue ethics furnishes us with a very useful way of addressing the justification of public health initiatives. How would the virtuous public health physician respond to a public health policy proposal? Is one's response too extreme, too much in favour of the individual, or of the community? Has this proposal been considered on its own merits, or have conclusions about other, seemingly similar proposals been unthinkingly assumed? What virtues are relevant to the situation, and what does their application amount to, practically speaking? Nonetheless, it would be an exaggeration to reduce public health ethics to the application of virtue ethics. The main reason for this is that more than one virtue is relevant in complex moral situations. Hence, in moral philosophy an important discussion about the virtues concerns whether there is one list of the 'correct' virtues that are salient at all times and places, which can be ranked or structured in such a way as to avoid clashes of virtue. The problem arises in the public health context, too. Dilemmas of the kind central to public health ethics typically involve numerous important virtues, some of which point in different directions. So, decisions have to be taken as to which virtue to base public health ethics judgements on. Consequently, virtue ethics should be acknowledged as a very useful resource, but it would be a mistake to rely on it exclusively in public health ethics, just as it would be unwise to base public health ethics solely on utilitarianism, Kantianism, principlism or any other single moral theory. (For more details – and a sceptical view – on virtue ethics in applied ethics, see Holland, 2010b, 2011, 2012b.)

Concluding remarks

The naïve utilitarian view of public health is that public health interventions are morally justified because they produce utility. This chapter has explained the main non-consequentialist grounds for resisting this view. Three non-consequentialist considerations are relevant. A public health intervention that offers substantial population health gain might, nonetheless, be dubious because of the kind of action it is, because it flouts some important principles of public health ethics, and/ or because it lacks virtue. As was the case in Chapter 1, this suggests three strategies for ethical analysis in public health. Of a proposed public health intervention we can ask whether it is, or involves, an action that is morally wrong by its very nature. For example, does it use people as mere means rather than ends-in-themselves? Second, we can ask whether it involves flouting important principles of public health ethics. For example, does it flout Upshur's principle of least restrictive or coercive means? Third, we can ask whether it expresses or ignores virtues important in public health. For example, does the proposal burden members of the target population for the sake of political expediency?

3 Liberal Political Philosophy

The previous two chapters introduced moral philosophy relevant to public health ethics, by presenting consequentialist and non-consequentialist rejoinders to the naïve view that any successful public health intervention is morally justified by utilitarianism. This chapter and the next take us further down the same road by stepping beyond moral philosophy and into political philosophy. Central to these chapters is what will be called the liberal objection to public health intervention, so we begin by introducing and explaining this. The present chapter then pursues the strategy of staying within the liberal tradition to see what resources are available to a liberal to meet the liberal objection to public health intervention. Two sorts of resources are discussed. The first appeals to Mill's harm principle. The second involves addressing what freedom is and invokes the concept of positive freedom. In the next chapter we widen the focus to look at responses to the liberal objection from beyond traditional liberalism.

Liberalism and the liberal objection

To introduce the liberal objection to public health intervention we need, first, to explain the political philosophy from which it emanates, namely, liberalism. This might seem an onerous task, for two reasons.

First, there is far too large a literature on liberalism to provide a comprehensive survey here; second, it is well known that political philosophy is one of those academic disciplines in which key terms are both ill-defined and used differently by different writers (Ryan 1993; Swift 2001: 51ff.). But things are not as bleak as this suggests because liberalism is 'a basic moral view on social life; one, moreover, that happens to be dominant in contemporary [Western] society' (Zwart 1999: 31). In other words, a broad brush stroke depiction of liberalism is not so hard because it is our '*de facto* political ideology' (Gostin 2003: 1141), the one that provides the political-philosophical backdrop to our everyday lives.

A good place to break into the circle of liberal ideas is to look a little more closely at a concept we have already encountered, namely, autonomy. The *Oxford English Dictionary* defines 'autonomy' as 'self-government; personal freedom'. The philosophical underpinnings of the principle of autonomy are in the Enlightenment emphasis on our capacity for rational self-governance, i.e., the view that persons are distinctive, and distinctively valuable, because they are rational creatures capable of bringing themselves under control, unlike mere animals which act instinctually. This view has become established as a major element in Western moral and political culture. It underpins the liberal emphasis on the rights of individuals, specifically the right of the individual to pursue their own conception of the good. A 'conception of the good' is a view of how to live based on one's beliefs about what makes life valuable or worthwhile. To pursue one's conception of the good requires freedom. Hence, the freedom or liberty – we can use these terms interchangeably – of the individual to be self-determining is considered by liberals to be pre-eminent.

Self-determining individuals can express their autonomy only if they are free from two things. First, they must be free from paternal influence. Paternalism is defined as follows: 'Practices and actions are paternalistic when those in positions of authority refuse to act according to people's wishes, or they restrict people's freedom, or in other ways attempt to influence their behavior, allegedly in the recipients' own best interests' (Häyry 1998: 449; see also Holland 2009). Hence, liberalism is an anti-paternalistic political philosophy (cf. Beauchamp 1985). Second, the liberal emphasis on autonomy and the rights of individuals to self-determination has profound implications for the kind of government, and the kind of relationship between the State and the citizenry, that can be considered legitimate. Liberals endorse State neutrality, i.e., the view that it is not legitimate for the State to make and enforce judgements about how individuals should live their lives. Correlatively, they are suspicious of State perfectionism, i.e., the view that some conceptions of the good are better than others and it is legitimate for the State to promote these. Quite where a liberal would stand on these matters will depend; for example, libertarianism is the form of liberalism that is most extreme in its emphasis on the right to freedom of individuals and State neutrality.

In sum, liberalism is an ideology to which the right of the individual to self-determination is central. It is easy to see that the liberal might be generally suspicious of public health: 'The most obvious distinction between public health and liberalism is public health's assertion that the health of a population is an objective good, measurable by objective criteria (i.e., morbidity, longevity, etc.), and not simply a matter of choice or preference' (Parmet 2003: 1234). It is also easy to see that the liberal, given their preference for State neutrality, might be hostile to specific, liberty-limiting, State-backed public health interventions. The upshot is the liberal objection.

The liberal objection

The liberal objection is a type of argument familiar from everyday experience and conversations about public health, and, most notably, from media coverage of public health policy. The objection – based on the fact that 'antipathy to government constraints on personal liberty runs deep' (Budetti 2001: 72) – is that such-and-such a public health policy is objectionable because it amounts to State interference in personal freedoms. For example, public health legislation banning smoking in public places is said to be objectionable because it would compromise smokers' freedom of choice; compulsory childhood immunization is objected to on the grounds that it transgresses parental rights to be free to decide what is best for their children; and objection to testing would-be immigrants for HIV is grounded in the claim that it would curtail the freedom of the individual to decline to consent to a medical intervention.

As is clear from these examples, different kinds of personal freedoms are said to be at stake and threatened by the various public health initiatives to which liberal objections are made. But whatever guise the liberal objection takes, it is a counter to naïve utilitarianism in public health. In other words, the naïve utilitarian view is that public health interventions are morally justified on utilitarian grounds; the liberal objection is that, on the contrary, such interventions are, or can be, dubious because they infringe on personal freedoms.

The liberal objection seems like a strong antidote to a naïve utilitarian approach to public health. But, in fact, once we dig a little deeper, it transpires that there are important rejoinders to it. This is not meant to imply that naïve utilitarianism was right for public health all along; rather, the point is that to evaluate properly the liberal objection involves discussing rejoinders to it. Hence, in the rest of this chapter we stay within the liberal tradition in order to identify features of liberalism itself which, when properly defined and applied, commit the liberal to allowing liberty-limiting State-backed public health interventions. Two such features come to mind, dealt with in turn in the rest of this chapter.

Liberalism and Mill's harm principle

In this section we consider a rejoinder to the liberal objection from within the liberal tradition. To work into this, it is useful to emphasize that liberalism is not anarchy. It is not the 'anything goes' view that no government is better than any government. Rather, liberals are concerned to do justice to their ideology by clearly delimiting the extent to which State interference in individual liberty is legitimate. Famously, this centres on Mill's harm or liberty principle, which is pivotal in the classical liberal tradition.

The harm principle

Since it is referred to a number of times in this book, it is worth citing the crucial passage in the writings of J.S. Mill at some length:

> The object of this Essay is to assert one very simple principle, as entitled to govern absolutely the dealings of society with the individual in the way of compulsion and control, whether the means used be physical force in the form of legal penalties, or the moral coercion of public opinion. That principle is, that the sole end for which mankind are warranted, individually or collectively, in interfering with the liberty of action of any of their number, is self-protection. That the only purpose for which power can be rightfully exercised over any member of a civilized community, against his will, is to prevent harm to others. His own good, either physical or moral, is not a sufficient warrant. He cannot rightfully be compelled to do or forbear because it will be better for him to do so, because it will make him happier, because, in the opinions of others, to do so would be wise, or even right. These are good reasons

for remonstrating with him, or reasoning with him, or persuading him, or entreating him, but not for compelling him, or visiting him with any evil in case he do otherwise. To justify that, the conduct from which it is desired to deter him must be calculated to produce evil to some one else. The only part of the conduct of any one, for which he is amenable to society, is that which concerns others. In the part which merely concerns himself, his independence is, of right, absolute. Over himself, over his own body and mind, the individual is sovereign. (Mill 1975: 14–15)

Before looking at how Mill's principle applies in public health, let's pause to clarify quite what it states. The key is to make two distinctions between types of actions. The first distinction is between actions that affect oneself and actions that affect others. The second is between actions that cause harm and those that create benefit. So, there are four kinds of actions: actions that (a) benefit oneself, (b) benefit others, (c) harm oneself and (d) harm others. And Mill's 'simple principle' – his harm, or liberty, principle – is that the State is within its rights to interfere with the liberty of individuals, or coerce them against their will, to avoid (d) actions that harm others. It might well be regrettable that an autonomous agent decides to eschew (a) and (b), or to go in for (c), but it would not be legitimate for the State to intervene in such cases.

Some initial clarificatory points about the harm principle are worth making. First, Mill was principally concerned with the limits to the legitimacy of State legislation, i.e., the extent to which the State can legislate against the free choices of autonomous individuals. As Gostin (2000: 18) puts it: 'Governments are formed not only to attend to the general needs of their constituents, but to insist, through force of law if necessary, that individuals and businesses act in ways that do not place others at unreasonable risk of harm.' But Mill was also concerned with the tyranny of moralizing and public opinion, i.e., with whether and when it is permissible for the moral majority to pressurize an individual to act against their will. Note, too, a strong necessity condition on the principle: State interference must be necessary to avoid (d) actions that harm others, in the sense that other less restrictive means are not available. Another detail is that the principle invites distinctions between types of third-party harms. We discuss this in more depth later; at this point it is enough to note that people can harm each other in quite different ways, ranging from outright physical harm to non-physical offences such as insults, and moral harms such as transgressing another's rights. Related to this is a rather deeper question about the moral neutrality of harm. The point here is that the concept of harm used in the principle is supposed to be morally neutral, otherwise it is question-begging to base the morality of limiting liberties on it; but it is hard to see what are considered to be harms as anything other than a function of the moral views extant in society.

The interpretation of the harm principle continues to be a controversial matter. In particular, the principle is often interpreted more expansively than has been presented so far, because Mill endorsed state actions aimed at getting people to benefit – not just avoid harms to – others (i.e., (b) above). For example, Mill (p. 16) states that one can be compelled to perform 'positive acts for the benefit of others'. Arguably, contemporary liberals should endorse a more expansive interpretation of the principle, not least because it is difficult to maintain the distinction between harming and benefiting. For example, should carriers be forcibly isolated during outbreaks because not doing so harms others, or because doing so benefits others? Here, we can put aside such interpretive issues because even on more expansive interpretations of the principle, it does not justify State paternalism (i.e., it does not permit governments to make people (a) benefit oneself).

Applying the harm principle in public health ethics

Notwithstanding these philosophical niceties, the crucial question for our purposes centres on how Mill's harm principle applies to the ethics of public health interventions. There will be occasions later in this book to apply the principle in some detail, so here a general description of how the harm principle works in public health ethics will suffice. A typical dialectic goes as follows. First, a public health initiative is mooted because it is expected to produce utility in the form of population health protection and promotion. Then the liberal objection is made that the initiative is an infringement on individual liberties. Finally, a rejoinder to the liberal objection is provided, to the effect that the infringement is justified on the grounds that, if implemented, the initiative will succeed in avoiding harm to third parties.

A classic example is the furore over banning smoking in public places. *Prima facie*, this is an illiberal policy. Fully autonomous agents who decide to smoke have the right to be free to do so. That giving up smoking would (a) benefit smokers and (c) avoid harm to smokers are, according to Mill's principle, dubious grounds for interfering in their 'liberty of action'. Hence the liberal objection to the ban. But then the rejoinder: the grounds for the ban are (d) to avoid third-party harm. Specifically, the public health problem addressed by the ban is said to be the ill effects of passive smoking; the ban is there to protect non-smokers in general, and bar and restaurant employees in particular, from the harm smokers cause them. So, the liberal ought to support this forceful public health policy on the grounds of protecting third parties.

Typically, this kind of dialectic continues in two directions. First, a conversation ensues about whether the public health initiative really does address third-party harms. The smoking ban is not so well suited to illustrate this because the epidemiology of passive smoking is relatively uncontentious. Better examples involve the rather nebulous harm to others of creating an economic burden. A case in point recalls the illustrative case study, used in previous chapters, of refusing to treat recalcitrant smokers. The liberal objection is that this is an assault on the individual's right to pursue a conception of the good that includes smoking. The rejoinder is that the recalcitrant smoker is causing third-party harm by selfishly using up scarce health care resources that could have helped others; so, the intervention is justified on Mill's harm principle. This is part of the more general question, addressed in Chapter 7, of whether it is legitimate for the State to interfere to change one's freely chosen unhealthy lifestyle, on the grounds that it creates a health economic burden to others. The appeal to Mill here is debatable because it is not obvious that this is the kind of third-party harm he had in mind. For one thing, the smoker can say that the harm is not caused by their actions, but by the failure of others to provide sufficient funding to cover everyone's health needs.

The other direction in which the dialectic continues concerns the *prima facie* nature of this kind of justification for liberty-limiting State interference. Let's assume that a public health intervention that impinges on individual freedoms would protect third parties. This is not a moral trump card; rather, it is one of a number of powerful but overridable considerations. Specifically, it may be that the third-party harm in question is not sufficiently serious to warrant the infringement. Good examples involve the harm of putting third parties at increased risk; what kind of, and how much, risk to others – as opposed to actual harm – is required for serious infringements on civil liberties to be justified? We revisit this in the discussion of the ethics of immunization in Chapter 9. Another good example involves a paradigmatic case of infringing on personal liberty for the sake of public health: at what point is risk to others sufficient to justify the invasive public health measure of quarantining?

Freedom: positive and negative conceptions

In this section we consider another rejoinder to the liberal objection to public health interventions, again from within the liberal tradition, one that requires looking more closely at what liberals mean by freedom. To begin, recall that the liberal objection to public health interventions is that they infringe on personal freedom by stopping people from pursuing their choices. For example, banning smoking in public places is said to be objectionable because it infringes on the smoker's freedom to choose to smoke. Importantly, there is a definition or conception or understanding of freedom implicit in this argument. Specifically, the liberal objection assumes that freedom is absence of constraint; i.e., one is free when there are no constraints, and unfree when there are constraints, on the pursuit of one's choices. The smoking ban, for example, is objected to because it undermines personal freedom by presenting a legal constraint on smokers. This account of freedom is known as the negative conception of freedom because it defines freedom as the absence of something, i.e., as the absence of constraint. The negative conception is an important, viable and respectable account of freedom. But, crucially, it is not the only one. There are various positive conceptions of freedom. Furthermore, some of them are at least as convincing as the negative account of freedom as the absence of constraints. Liberal objections to public health intervention – i.e., that such-and-such an intervention is an objectionable infringement on personal liberty – appear quite differently on some positive conceptions of freedom.

Before getting further into the details, let's pause to get a feel for the basic distinction between negative and positive conceptions of freedom, and what motivates the latter. Is the homeless person I passed on the way to work this morning free to fly to France today? The answer is, yes and no, depending on what you mean by 'free'. On the one hand, nothing and nobody is stopping them. For example, there are no laws stopping them, a UK citizen, from entering France, no one is going to take it upon themselves to physically obstruct them, and so on. Since there are no actual constraints on their flying off to France, and given the negative conception of freedom as the absence of constraint, they are perfectly at liberty to do so. But, of course, in another sense they are obviously far from free to fly to France. The homeless person quite lacks the means to do this, not least because they do not have enough money to buy the plane ticket. So, if freedom is construed negatively as freedom from constraint, obstruction or interference, the homeless person is free to fly to France. But if freedom is construed positively as, roughly, the freedom to do things, then they are not free to fly to France.

The background to this general distinction between negative and positive conceptions of freedom is one of the most famous essays in political philosophy, 'Two concepts of liberty' by Isaiah Berlin (1969). Berlin's main point – that the negative conception of liberty is preferable to the positive, because the latter is dangerous and underpins totalitarianism – need not detain us at this point; nor does most of the subsequent discussion of Berlin's position. But one point is worth clarifying. It was very natural in the previous paragraph – and it used to be standard – to explain the basic negative/positive freedom distinction in terms of 'freedom from ...' versus 'freedom to ...'. In other words, one has the negative freedom to do X if one is free from constraints on doing X, and positive freedom is a matter of being able to do X. But, although useful by way of introduction, this is not a good way to express the distinction. The problem is that all freedoms are both 'freedoms from' and 'freedoms to'. For example, I am free to use my university's library both because I am free from obstructions to using it, and 'free to' in that I have the appropriate membership. Given this, it is typical for political philosophers to retain the intuitive appeal of the negative/positive freedom distinction, but not in terms of 'freedom from ...' versus 'freedom to ...'.

Swift's (2001: 51–68) way of going about this is particularly clear and informative. Swift explains three distinctions between types or conceptions of freedom that inform the negative/positive freedom distinction whilst avoiding the simplistic 'freedom from ...' versus 'freedom to ...' formula. Each of his three distinctions includes a viable positive conception of freedom. His third distinction is between freedom as political participation versus freedom beginning where politics ends. Since this is not so relevant for our purposes, it can be ignored here. But his other two distinctions are very pertinent. Let's explain each, and then see how they help to justify public health intervention.

Effective freedom

Swift's first distinction is between effective freedom and formal freedom. Swift defines this as follows: 'The difference between effective and formal freedom is the difference between having the power or capacity to act in a certain way and the mere absence of interference' (p. 55). This definition makes the distinction sound very close to the dubious 'freedom from ...' versus 'freedom to ...' formula. Be that as it may, the point is that we have here a credible notion of positive freedom: 'People's real or effective (or, sometimes, "positive") freedom can be promoted not just by leaving them alone, but by putting them in a position to do things they would not otherwise be able to do' (p. 56). Importantly for our purposes, Swift illustrates this as follows:

> Think about somebody who is very ill, and cannot pursue her preferred career without medical treatment. If freedom were merely absence of interference by others, we would have to say that she is free to pursue that career – she simply lacks the effective capacity (here health) to do it. Armed with the distinction between formal and effective freedom we could ... say that while nobody is preventing her from pursuing that career, so she is formally free to do so, she will not have the effective freedom to pursue it unless she is given the medical treatment. Here is [an] example where the distinction between formal and effective freedom looks capable of doing some work, and where the state might be thought able to act to promote the effective freedom of some of its citizens (in this case by providing medical care). (P. 59)

This sounds eminently reasonable: State provision of health care is justified on the grounds that it promotes freedom construed positively as effective freedom. But the thought naturally occurs that we can push this idea further. Note Swift's final comment that 'the state might be thought able to act to promote the effective freedom of some of its citizens (in this case by providing medical care)'. Although it is uncontentious, it seems odd to restrict the conclusion to the argument about effective freedom to permissibility, i.e., to what the State is permitted or allowed to do. Surely we might go further to talk about an obligation here: the State has the *prima facie* obligation or duty to provide the protagonist with the medical care in question. Of course, this is only *prima facie* because there are many considerations that might rule the medical intervention out, such as a lack of health care resources. Nonetheless, it seems sensible to say that one of the duties of the State is to promote the freedom of its citizens, effective freedom is a viable positive account of freedom, the medical care in question would promote effective freedom, therefore, all other things being equal, the State ought to provide it (and, conversely, the woman has a right to it).

But if this is right, we can go further still. For the sake of argument, suppose that the protagonist in Swift's example has angina caused by smoking, the medical care being a coronary bypass. According to the previous argument, the State has a *prima facie* obligation to provide the surgery, and the patient a right to it, on the grounds that it would increase their effective freedom. But then, arguably, it is permissible by the same token to implement policies aimed at getting them to quit smoking in the first place. This is simply a matter of consistency: if creating effective freedom grounds rights and obligations concerning medical treatment, creating effective freedom can ground attempts to prevent the condition requiring treatment in the first place. Policies such as banning smoking in public places, aggressive health communication campaigns such as fear messages intended to shock smokers into giving up, 'sin taxing' cigarettes, and such like, are all justified on the same grounds: they aim at protecting and enhancing the effective freedom of citizens.

The point is that intrusive public health interventions that undermine people's negative freedom – because the interventions in question provide constraints – can still be justified on the liberal grounds that they promote freedom construed positively as effective freedom. Of course, much more needs to be said, and there is space here to pursue this only a little further. Here is one version of how a subsequent debate might unfold. An advocate of the liberal objection might respond to the appeal to effective freedom by pointing out that the protagonist in Swift's example is a patient whose effective freedom has been curtailed by her illness; by contrast, public health is typically aimed at asymptomatic populations who have plenty of effective freedom, but whose negative freedom (i.e., freedom as absence of constraint) will be reduced by the interventions in question. In other words, it is one thing to say that Swift's protagonist ought to be treated in order to restore her effective freedom, but another to say that the negative freedom of healthy smokers should be compromised by interventions that aim at helping some of them to avoid the loss of effective freedom in the future. Roughly, the point is, why should a healthy smoker lose (negative) freedom now, on the off-chance that doing so will avoid their losing (positive) freedom in the future?

A proponent of public health intervention might respond by suggesting that the question is somewhat naïve. It is natural to take one's health for granted. Health is a necessary condition for effective freedom. So, it is natural to take one's effective freedom for granted. But the fact is that the best way to compromise one's effective freedom is to get ill. Any debilitating illness – ranging from the relatively inconvenient, such as flu, to the very severe, such as lung cancer – seriously compromises one's freedom construed positively as effective freedom.

By contrast, the right to be (negatively) free from constraint to smoke seems trivial. So, from the public health perspective, as far as freedoms are concerned, the important one is to stay healthy and enjoy effective freedom, as opposed to cherishing one's rather paltry negative freedoms, such as the freedom to smoke.

But, of course, this dialogue can be continued. Advocates of the liberal objection can appeal to various factors, such as the questionable evidence base for many preventive interventions that compromise negative freedom, the role of addiction in some of the relevant debates, such as the one about banning smoking in public places, and so on. Rather than pursue this dialogue further here, let's turn to Swift's other relevant positive construal of freedom.

Freedom as autonomy

Swift (pp. 59–64) distinguishes freedom as autonomy from freedom as doing what one wants. The former – freedom as autonomy – is another plausible positive conception of freedom. We have encountered the notion of autonomy various times already. The basic idea – and literal definition – of autonomy is self-rule, i.e., one's ability to be in control of, or govern, oneself. So, if autonomy is self-rule, and freedom is autonomy, then one is free if, and to the extent that, one is in control of, or governs, oneself. So, someone who does what they want may or may not be acting autonomously. This is because they might well be fulfilling their wants and desires, but not in such a way that they are really in control of, or governing, themselves. A clear, simple example is addictive behaviour. The addict who reaches for the bottle or another shot might well be doing what they want, or be fulfilling their present desires, but their autonomy, their capacity for self-rule, is compromised by their addiction. So, they are free in one (negative) sense, unfree in another (positive) sense:

> Our idea of the autonomous person seems to involve more than just the capacity to act on particular desires and choices. It suggests a more general capacity to be self-determining, to be in control of one's own life. (Norman 2005: 72)

Two points of clarification about the basic idea of freedom as autonomy can be made. First, whilst freedom as autonomy and effective freedom – as discussed in the previous subsection – both construe freedom positively, they are completely different from one another. Recall that Swift explains effective freedom in terms of 'power or capacity to act in a certain way' and being 'in a position to do things they would not otherwise be able to do'. By contrast, freedom as autonomy is not about being facilitated or enabled to act, but about whether one's actions emanate from self-rule or merely as the upshot of present wants and desires. The second clarificatory point is that it is very contentious to define freedom as autonomy. This is because it requires us to say of people who act as they want that they are not really free because they did not act autonomously. It requires us to distinguish between people who are doing what they really want as opposed to what they merely happen to desire. But who is the 'us' making such a decision? And on what grounds? There seems to be a lot of scope for abuse here, as the moral majority castigates people for acting in ways it happens not to favour.

Nonetheless, for all its contentiousness, the notion of freedom as autonomy – as opposed to merely doing what one happens to want – has intuitive appeal and applies well to certain kinds of public health interventions. The best examples are health education and health communication campaigns, because there is an obvious connection between autonomy, ignorance and education. Suppose someone wants to smoke because they like the taste and the social effects, and are quite unaware of the health risks. If freedom is construed as doing what one wants then they are acting freely. But they are not acting autonomously because they lack the information required to make properly informed, rational decisions. Public health interventions aimed at providing the required information about health behaviours and risks are justified on the grounds that they increase freedom as autonomy. In sum, if freedom is autonomy, and autonomy requires health education and information, then public health campaigns aimed at informing people about risky health behaviours are justified.

However, as ever, more needs to be said. For one thing, this is really a rather limited application in public health of the idea of freedom as autonomy. Moreover, most people do not find purely informative health communication campaigns particularly objectionable. Objection strengthens the more aggressive the campaigns become, i.e., when they seem less about helping people to make properly autonomous decisions, and more about 'forcing' them to change their behaviours in ways approved of by public health officialdom. So, for example, people object more to price restructuring and 'sin taxing' fatty foods, and less to mere food labelling, because the former are seen as ways of forcing the 'right' decision out of people as opposed to inviting people to make it for themselves. Let's leave that dialogue here, and turn to a more general objection to the line of thought discussed in this section.

Liberalism and positive freedom

The general idea in this section is to stay within liberalism to argue that, whilst advocates of the liberal objection to public health tend to take a negative conception of freedom for granted, there are viable positive conceptions of freedom on which some liberty-limiting public health activities can be justified. That this line of thought can do some work in public health ethics has already been demonstrated. But it is not entirely persuasive. The problem is that liberals can dig in their heels by objecting to the very notion of positive freedom. They would do so because they think there is something inherently dangerous about going beyond the idea that protecting freedom means removing constraints on people (i.e., negative freedom). This worry has a strong tradition; for example, as mentioned above, the main point of Isaiah Berlin's famous essay is to endorse negative conceptions of freedom at the expense of positive ones, precisely because of the latter's association with perfectionism and totalitarianism. So, the general problem is that liberals can dig in their heels to resist the liberty-limiting appeal to positive conceptions of freedom.

One thing that mitigates this problem is that there are different ways of construing freedom positively. The liberal should pause to distinguish amongst these to see how strongly they object to them. This can be demonstrated by reference to the two ways of construing freedom considered in this section, i.e., effective freedom and freedom as autonomy. Arguably, liberals should respond differently to these. They will certainly worry about freedom as autonomy. Creating autonomy seems to require a vision of the autonomous agent as a certain kind of person, one who likes, wants and desires certain things, who tends to choose in certain ways. Liberals will find this is at best patronizing, and at worst just the kind of health fascism and State nannying that concerned them about public health in the first place. Social engineering in the name of freedom of this sort strikes liberals as particularly nefarious. But, on the other hand, liberals might be more sympathetic to the notion of effective freedom, because protecting and enhancing effective freedom is about enabling people to do what they themselves want, as opposed to what others say they really want. So, it seems plausible that some support for preventive health campaigns is provided by the fact that they promote effective freedom by enabling people to do more of what they want than they could otherwise.

Concluding remarks

This chapter has moved the discussion from moral to political philosophy. Liberalism and the liberal objection to public health intervention were introduced. Generally speaking, liberals are suspicious of public health interventions which threaten personal freedom. Two responses from within the liberal tradition were discussed. The first is Mill's famous harm principle: a liberal would endorse coercive public health measures which are intended to avoid third-party harms (more detailed applications of the harm principle to specific public health programmes are discussed in some of the case studies in Part II). The second centres on what freedom is: the liberal objection is based on the negative conception of freedom as absence of constraints, but two positive conceptions of freedom were presented to which a liberal can appeal when evaluating public health interventions.

4 Beyond Traditional Liberalism

The previous chapter considered responses to the liberal objection to public health intervention from within the liberal tradition. This chapter discusses two further responses that take us increasingly further away from the liberal mainstream. First, libertarian paternalism tries to combine the liberal's insistence on personal freedom with paternalistic public health interventions. This sounds oxymoronic but advocates argue not and, in fact, libertarian paternalism grounds a very influential approach to public policy, namely, 'nudging' people towards certain options, including healthy behaviour. In the second section of this chapter we move outside of liberalism altogether by looking at a non-liberal political theory, namely, communitarianism. Communitarians criticize liberalism for overemphasizing individual rights and freedoms at the expense of communal values and benefits; it is natural for public health advocates to appeal to communitarianism as a justification for curbing individual choice for the sake of population health.

Libertarian paternalism

As discussed in the previous chapter, Mill's harm principle is a major theoretical resource within the liberal tradition. The principle provides justification for public health coercion on grounds of avoiding third-party harms. The reach of the principle can be extended by interpreting harms expansively. For example, if risk of, as opposed to actual, harm is included – along with long-term and indirect harms, such as using up scarce health resources – more and more interventions are justifiable under the principle. But however expansively it is interpreted, Mill's principle rules out State paternalism, i.e., coercion by the State to get people to benefit themselves: 'His own good, either physical or moral, is not a sufficient warrant [for exercising power against someone's will].' Since the overall effect of getting each individual to improve their own health is better population health, this prohibition on State paternalism means that significant public health gains are lost. This is why the harm principle does not go far enough for some public health advocates.

The upshot is a dilemma: achieve public health goals by getting individuals to act in their own best health interests, but at the expense of liberal values; or preserve liberal values, but at the expense of public health gains that would be achieved by public health paternalism. Libertarian paternalism is designed to avoid this dilemma (Thaler and Sunstein 2003). We can think of libertarianism as a comparatively extreme form of liberalism that emphasizes the value of personal liberty and an individual's right to self-determination, the only side constraint being the obligation to respect everyone else's equal right to the same. Paternalism was introduced in the previous chapter; the defining characteristic of a paternalistic action is that it is intended to get someone else to act in their own best interests. Given this, 'libertarian paternalism' seems oxymoronic because the libertarian wants individuals to decide what is best for themselves whereas paternalists think they know what is in people's best interests (Mitchell 2005).

But libertarian paternalists argue that their approach is not oxymoronic (Sunstein and Thaler 2003). Libertarian paternalism is the theoretical basis of 'nudge' – the title of a seminal book by Thaler and Sunstein (2009) – which has become influential in public policy planning. Thaler and Sunstein appeal to behavioural sciences such as psychology and behavioural economics to show that people tend not to make rational choices in their own best interests because they are subject to irrational influences on their decisions. In particular, choosers are subject to cognitive biases such as default settings and the status quo bias: people are influenced by existing arrangements, as opposed to ignoring these and choosing the most rational option. Similarly, choosers are subject to what are known as 'choice-framing effects'; notably, the way in which options are presented influences people's decisions. For example, patients are more likely to choose a medical treatment when it is presented as having a 90 per cent chance of success than when it is presented as having a 10 per cent chance of failure.

Irrational influences on choosers are unavoidable because, for example, choice scenarios have to be arranged in some fashion and options have to be presented in some way or other. Sunstein and Thaler suggest that, since they are unavoidable anyway, it is sensible to utilize these irrational influences to get people to choose in their own best interests. After all, the alternative is to allow such influences to motivate people to choose sub-optimally, which seems perverse. So planners should design the 'choice architecture' – the structured circumstances in which choices are made – to nudge people towards rational options. This is paternalistic because it is getting people to choose in their own best interest. But it is acceptable to a libertarian because the cost of resisting a nudge is non-existent to very low (as a guide, libertarian paternalists recommend that it takes no more than the click of a computer mouse to resist a nudge). Hence, 'libertarian paternalism' is not oxymoronic.

An illustration will help to clarify the approach. Consider a café. Customers choose food from a variety of options. Their choices are susceptible to irrational influences. For example, how customers behave is affected by where options are placed (people are more likely to choose the options that are placed closer to hand). The café has to be arranged somehow so the influence of the layout of items is unavoidable. Libertarian paternalists advocate using such influences to nudge customers to choose in their own best interests, i.e., to select healthy items. After all, the alternative is to prompt customers to choose unhealthy options against their best interests. Constructing the choice architecture so as to nudge people towards the healthy options is paternalistic; but it is acceptable to a libertarian because the cost of resisting the nudge is no greater than, say, having to walk a little further for the unhealthy food.

Theoretical objections

Some general constraints on public health nudges will be suggested in the next subsection, and promising applications of the approach will be discussed in Part II. But first, let's consider theoretical objections to libertarian paternalism. Arguably, some of the most familiar criticisms of the approach are not as important as they seem. For example, the point is often made that libertarian paternalism is unoriginal because the influence of irrational factors on choices has long been known by marketing companies and advertising agencies (Marteau et al. 2011). In fact, it is not even an original approach to public policy planning; social marketing, for example, which aims at social goals by using techniques borrowed from the commercial sector, predates the nudge agenda (Ling et al. 1992). But it matters less that libertarian paternalism is original than whether it is politically and ethically acceptable, and practicable.

Similarly, nudging is often said to be ineffective (Salazar 2012). But the evidence here is incomplete. Nudging might take longer than has thus far been allowed, planners might get better at utilizing behavioural techniques, new techniques might be devised, or nudging might be effective in untried choice scenarios. Besides, the claim that nudging is practically ineffective is not an objection to the approach in principle, which leaves it open for nudges to be combined with other sorts of interventions as part of a mixed approach to behaviour change. This would not be problematic for a libertarian paternalist because no one advocates nudging as the only approach to getting people to choose more healthily.

A subtler version of this criticism is that the approach is of the wrong sort to be effective. Specifically, nudges are 'shallow' in only being intended to influence people's actual choices as opposed to the motivational sets from which their preferences emanate. For example, people might be nudged to eat less fatty food on specific occasions – as in the café example above – but become no more 'body aware' or health conscious, so quickly slip back into old habits. Another version of this charge is that nudges cannot be effective because they do not address underlying structural determinants of unhealthy behaviour and resultant health inequalities, such as economic disadvantage and social constraints. In fact, it is argued, when ramifications such as these are taken into account, nudging is not only ineffectual but, worse still, can result in a net negative effect.

The problem with this objection is that it begs the question as to what sort of public planning to allow. Libertarian paternalists advocate nudges precisely because they are 'shallow' in the sense that they are aimed at changing specific behaviour in discrete choice settings. Being libertarians, they would be very suspicious of allowing public planners to attempt something 'deeper', such as changing people's motivational sets or a society's social structures. This is because libertarians want to keep State intervention to a minimum in order to allow individuals the liberty to decide for themselves. So the very thing for which the approach is here being criticized – its shallowness – is a virtue according to the libertarian paternalist.

Another sort of objection is in the form of slippery slope arguments (Rizzo and Whitman 2009). The general structure of slippery slope arguments is: action A may seem permissible but it is at the top of a slippery slope to action B, which is impermissible. There are two versions of this sort of argument against libertarian paternalism, neither of which is convincing. The first is that nudges are the top of a slippery slope to a myriad of further nudges. This is certainly plausible; nudges might proliferate, for example because planners become psychologically predisposed to create more nudges as nudging becomes commonplace, or a nudge designed to address one sort of irrational influence on agents might necessitate further nudges to address a different irrational influence. But it is hard to see that what is at the bottom of this slippery slope is objectionable because it does not matter how many nudges there are – one or millions – so long as each nudge is very easy to resist.

According to the other version of the argument, what lies at the bottom of the slippery slope are objectionable interventions, i.e., coercive interventions:

> A fat tax helps the individual to improve his diet … However, he might also reduce his effort toward other subgoals, like exercise … As a result, policymakers have reason to intervene further – by increasing the fat tax, or subsidizing gym membership, or perhaps even resorting to food bans and exercise mandates. (Rizzo and Whitman 2009: 709)

But this is not a fair criticism because the whole point of libertarian paternalism is to rule out coercive interventions of the sort Rizzo and Whitman suggest. So long as planners understand this, there is no reason to think they will shift from nudging to coercion. Of course, planners might not understand this, and naïvely coerce people; but this would be a failing of planners, not of the nudge agenda.

So, familiar objections to libertarian paternalism do not seem to be very strong. But libertarians do have a legitimate concern about nudging which centres on the remit of the State. Libertarianism disallows a role for the State in devising and imposing a conception of the good – understood as a more or less comprehensive account of what is important in life and how it should be lived – and insists on each individual's right to devise and pursue their own conception of the good: 'Most importantly, the state does not impose any substantive notion of the good life but helps individuals retain freedom to determine their own preferred ends' (Mitchell 2005: 1263). So a State that nudges is objectionable to libertarians because it transgresses their strictures on how a conception of the good is devised and pursued: by individuals, says the libertarian, not by governments.

How strong is this objection that nudging gets the role of government wrong? One point is that there are disparate versions of libertarianism, some of which might allow State planning of the nudge variety. But it is hard to see how any theory that endorses a State's devising a conception of the good is properly called libertarianism. Perhaps State nudges are not based on anything as grand as a conception of the good, i.e., on anything as grand as an overview of how life should be lived. But nudges cannot be based on how people actually behave because the point of nudging is to change behaviour. Nor can they be based on how most people behave or on how people would choose if mandated to choose: the former would be a case of 'the tyranny of the majority'; libertarian paternalists expressly reject the latter for most choice scenarios.

The standard and oft-repeated libertarian paternalist's response to this sort of objection is that State planners base nudges not on how governments think people should live their lives but on what makes people better off *as judged by themselves*. But this might well seem disingenuous. How is it to be established that a nudge is what 'nudgees' themselves judge is best for themselves? When and how were they asked? Libertarian paternalists might appeal here to 'ideal deliberators'; i.e., what people themselves judge to be in their own best interest is what an ideal deliberator – who has full knowledge, plenty of time, high intelligence, etc. – would judge to be in their own best interest. But the sort of behavioural and lifestyle options towards which people are nudged are contestable even by ideal deliberators. For example, disputes about diet are not resolved by having more knowledge, time to deliberate, etc., because they are grounded in different conceptions of how to live one's life, such as whether to be health conscious and prudent or hedonistic and riotous.

So, a libertarian has a theoretical objection to libertarian paternalism. But this does not rule out public health nudges because public health is not a libertarian endeavour. The aim of public health is not liberty but protecting and promoting population health. Hence, even if the libertarian has a problem with nudging, public health planners might still consider it to be well suited to public health. This raises the question as to whether behavioural techniques advocated by libertarian paternalists are useful in achieving public health goals. Nudging seems like a promising way to ease the tension between the pursuit of public health goals and individuals' liberty – the theme of this book

– because it steers people towards healthy options without coercing them (Ménard 2010).

General constraints on public health nudges: uncertainty, criminality and addiction

The strategy for the rest of this section is to outline and criticize some suggested applications of libertarian paternalist techniques in the public health literature. This is not intended as an aggressive dismissal of the articles in question, all of which address important public health questions and make good points. Rather, the aim is to tease out some general constraints on public health nudges. Specifically, three conditions on libertarian paternalist strategies emerge from this discussion, centring on uncertainty, criminality and addiction.

First, Wheeler et al. (2011) apply libertarian paternalist strategies to prostate specific antigen (PSA) screening for prostate cancer. They describe two current decision-making approaches, informed and shared decision making (IDM and SDM), and suggest augmenting these with nudges to improve patients' decisions about, and ameliorate harms caused by, PSA screening. What makes this suggestion instructive is the uncertainty surrounding the screening programme. As Wheeler et al. explain, uncertainty arises at the population level because the best evidence as to whether the programme reduces rates of mortality is unclear. Uncertainty also arises at the individual level because screening can result in overdiagnosis and overtreatment which, in turn, cause serious unnecessary harms to individual patients, including incontinence and impotence.

Clinical uncertainty surrounding PSA persists despite clear consensus on values and goals, and impeccable medical expertise. Sometimes, medicine is simply too uncertain for anyone to know the best treatment plan. In a case such as PSA, clinical uncertainty renders it unclear as to what options are optimal: more screening, further testing and treatment, or to decline screening, testing and/or treatment. Given this, is it appropriate to augment IDM and SDM with libertarian paternalist strategies? The worry is that nudging is irrelevant because planners simply do not know which options to nudge patients towards. This suggests a general constraint on public health nudges: nudging is inappropriate in the context of the sort of deep clinical uncertainty illustrated by the PSA case. Given that public health is bedevilled by uncertainty, this is an important restriction on public health nudges.

To introduce a second constraint on public health nudges, consider that public health is State sanctioned and governed by legal strictures and law enforcement. Is it appropriate to employ libertarian paternalist strategies in areas of public health governed by legislation? Stevenson's (2006) discussion of the cocaine vaccine is instructive. The vaccine works when the anti-cocaine agent injected into the bloodstream bonds with cocaine molecules to form a compound too big to pass through the blood–brain barrier, so it does not afford the user any pleasurable experiences. Given this, there is no point in buying cocaine and the drug is rendered non-addictive. Stevenson considers four applications of the cocaine vaccine: vaccinating parolees or those with a history of drug abuse; vaccinating welfare recipients; universal vaccination; vaccinating air traffic controllers. He pursues the research question as to whether the 'Sunstein/Thaler model' of libertarian paternalism is appropriate to each of these four applications. It is worth pointing out that Stevenson seems to have in mind mandatory vaccinations of the groups he discusses (parolees, welfare recipients, etc.), a typical suggestion being that 'Sunstein/Thaler's model would allow for mandatory vaccinations for this group'. There seems to be a category error here because the point of 'Sunstein/Thaler's model' is to get people to choose freely what is in their best interests as opposed to mandatory interventions. Libertarian paternalism in this context would advocate nudging people to get vaccinated whilst allowing them to remain free not to do so, which disallows 'mandatory vaccinations'. Similarly, some of the policies Stevenson considers make the cost of choosing the suboptimal option so high as to rule out calling them nudges. For example, if the cost of refusing the cocaine vaccine is one's parole or welfare benefits, choosers are more than nudged to get vaccinated, so the strategy would not be endorsed by libertarian paternalists.

Furthermore, at various points Stevenson seems to adopt approaches that are alternatives to libertarian paternalism. For example, he deploys 'utilitarian arguments', such as that utility would be maximized by inoculating young people against the attractions of drugs. And the harm principle is clearly at work. This is most notable in his discussion of vaccinating air traffic controllers, a 'somewhat randomly' selected example of professionals whose decisions involve 'high stakes ... hundreds of lives may be at stake in each of [their] decisions' (p. 12). As this description suggests, policies such as compulsory drugs testing and mandatory vaccination are justified by the need to avoid third-party harms, not by the need to get air traffic controllers to choose in their own best interests without coercing them.

Notwithstanding this, Stevenson's discussion remains illustrative. One thing that makes the applications of libertarian paternalist strategies to the cocaine vaccine contentious is that the principal options – purchasing, possessing and using cocaine – are illegal. This is obviously dissimilar to paradigmatic nudges, such as getting people to choose healthy meals in a café, where all relevant options are legally permitted. Is it appropriate to deploy libertarian paternalist strategies in choice scenarios in which principal options have been criminalized? Arguably not, because the point of libertarian paternalism is to nudge people to choose certain options whilst remaining free to do otherwise, whereas agents are and should be coerced to decline – not left at liberty to choose – criminal options. This suggests another general constraint on nudging: libertarian paternalist strategies are inappropriate to choices governed by public health law.

To introduce a third constraint on public health nudges, note that a major theme in public health includes abstinence policies, cessation services and harm reduction strategies aimed at unhealthy behaviour involving addictive substances. Is nudging appropriate in the context of addictive behaviour? An obvious worry is that nudging will not work for substance users because the relevant behavioural techniques – choice framing, default setting, etc. – are too subtle: they will be overwhelmed by the urge to satisfy cravings which is characteristic of addictive behaviour. But this might be too quick. Addictive behaviour is rational on some models of addiction, which might salvage the libertarian paternalist approach by suggesting that addicts retain sufficient autonomy to be susceptible to the influence of nudges (see, for example, Becker and Murphy 1988).

But rational addiction models are usually based on evidence such as that substance users are price sensitive (for example, drug users' purchasing patterns change in response to increases in costs of drugs). This might well ground some approaches to addictive behaviour modification, such as heavily sin taxing a substance. But these are economic levers that exploit agents' economic rationality, as opposed to nudges which appeal to the non-rational part of people's natures and which can be resisted without significant economic (or other) costs. So the libertarian paternalist approach is not salvaged by endorsing rational addiction models.

Furthermore, from a public health perspective nudging is inappropriate to addictive behaviour because other sorts of interventions are more important. People addicted to substances such as drugs, alcohol and tobacco need complex and carefully constructed programmes drawing on various disciplines including addiction studies and health psychology. Nudging seems simply irrelevant to this. This same line of thought applies to public health programmes aimed at maintaining and promoting mental health, because mental illness often manifests in compulsive behaviour. The same points apply: nudges are ineffective ways of influencing the compulsive behaviour of people with mental health problems; and other sorts of interventions – ranging from pharmaceutical through cognitive-behavioural to 'talking therapies' – are more important. The upshot is another general constraint: libertarian paternalist strategies are inappropriate when the choice setting involves addictive or otherwise compulsive behaviour.

To sum up this discussion, nudging is a promising way of achieving public health goals but we should be alert to some general constraints. Three have been suggested here: nudging is inappropriate given uncertainty, criminality or addiction. But less controversial applications of the approach might well be both effective and politically more acceptable than heavy-handed, Draconian interventions. This is pursued Chapter 7, where the general issue of behaviour modification for the sake of health promotion is discussed. (For a more detailed version of this discussion of libertarian paternalism, see Holland 2014.)

Non-liberal political philosophy: communitarianism

This section discusses a final response to the liberal objection to public health interventions that they infringe on personal freedoms. Since this objection is grounded in liberalism, an obvious strategy is to question whether liberalism is an adequate political philosophy in the first place. This introduces communitarianism, a different political philosophy that has developed out of a forceful critique of liberalism. There has been much interest in applying communitarianism in public health ethics debates, either explicitly or implicitly, in order to counter the assumption that the liberal objection is well grounded. The aim of this section is to introduce the communitarian critique of liberalism, illustrate how it informs public health ethics, and discuss how compelling the appeal to communitarianism is in debates about public health intervention.

The best way to introduce communitarianism is to get a feel for what is at stake between liberal and communitarian political philosophies. Consider a continuum from a more individualistic-minded to more community-minded attitude. At the first pole, people think that what matters are things such as individuality, individual rights, personal autonomy, freedom of choice, freedom from Draconian constraints by the government, and such like. At the other pole, people think that what matters are things like membership of communities (including nuclear and extended families, neighbourhoods, towns, States and associations), being similar to others, sharing interests, accepting responsibility for one another, leading interconnected lives, and so on. The point of the communitarian critique is that liberalism overemphasizes the former set of features, in particular the individual and their freedom to live as they choose. This overemphasis in the liberal tradition on the individual's freedom to pursue their own conception of the good has resulted in neglect of various goods and values that belong under the umbrella notion of community. Communitarians argue that the community is, and should be, at the centre of our moral thinking. By emphasizing the social nature of our life, identity, relationships and institutions, the communitarian aims to restore the notion of community to proper prominence.

The communitarian critique: some details

Having got a feel for what is at stake in the liberalism–communitarianism debate, we need to move on to some of the details. Let's start by clarifying the precise target of the communitarian critique. This might seem unproblematic: communitarians are against liberalism. But this is too simplistic because 'liberalism is a broad umbrella, which encompasses not only George W. Bush ... and Ralph Nader, but also Immanuel Kant, John Stuart Mill, Ronald Dworkin and John Rawls, as well as innumerable other theorists' (Parmet 2003: 1223). Nonetheless, there is one idea, basic to liberalism and shared by all members of the liberal tradition, to which communitarians object. This is the idea that people are best thought of as individual, atomistic, unembedded, self-standing, rational and autonomous choosers. Whatever else Parmet's 'innumerable theorists' disagree about, liberals subscribe to this, their defining view of people or 'conception of the self'. We encountered this view in the previous section: pre-eminent for the liberal of any hue is the protection (from, for example, paternalism) of the individual's right to freely pursue their own conception of the good. Communitarians object to this, and 'criticize individualists for conceiving of human beings in terms of radically disembodied subjects, as *free choosers*' (M. Parker 1998: 17; see also Raeder 1998).

How do communitarians criticize this liberal conception of people as 'free choosers'? It is tempting to think that the communitarian simply does not like liberalism's emphasis on individuals and their freedom, and that they prefer the idea of community and all the rather homely virtues – support, mutual co-operation, and so on – that it implies. This is a mistake, because the communitarian critique is much more tough-minded. In fact, communitarians think that the liberal view of people is incoherent: 'To imagine a person incapable of constructive attachments ... is not to conceive an ideally free and rational agent, but to imagine a person wholly without character, without moral depth' (Sandel 1982: 179). To clarify, the incoherence is this. Liberals depict people as both free-floating ('disembodied', to use Parker's metaphor) individuals and 'choosers'. But only people with fully formed characters and moral depth can genuinely choose anything, from a general conception of the good to specific options presented in specific circumstances. One acquires the requisite character and depth by being initiated into the culture or tradition maintained by one's community. So, the very thing the liberal emphasizes in order to defend – namely, free choice – entails that people are not as the liberal depicts them, i.e., 'disembodied'. In sum, communitarians 'locate the very possibility of being an individual within particular societies, cultures or communities' (Brecher 1999: 610; see, also, Walzer 1990; Kymlicka 1990, 1993; Avineri and de-Shalit 1992).

Communitarianism in public health ethics

This appeal to communitarianism is strikingly frequent in public health debates. For example, Zwart (1999) contrasts 'liberal and communitarian views on the allocation of health care resources'. Rothstein's (2004) important analysis of 'traditional' responses to the SARS outbreak of 2002–3 is based on the following contrast:

> The countries most affected by SARS are known for their communitarian values. The United States, which was largely spared the SARS epidemic – and which may not be so fortunate in the future – is known more for libertarian values. (Pp. 175–6)

Along similar lines, Cribb and Duncan (2002: 61ff.), in exploring the ethics of sexual health promotion in general, ask whether teenage pregnancy services in particular are in the interests of individuals or communities. Brecher (1999) applies liberal and communitarian conceptions of medical need to the management of organ transplantation, arguing, for example, that, since 'communities are characteristically trans-generational entities', an individual does not cease to be bound to their community and the needs of its members even after death.

And, in a series of influential works, Gostin (2002b, 2003) has discussed the ethics of the public health response to the threat of bioterrorism in terms of the debate between liberalism and communitarianism (cf. Annas 2002; Sidel et al. 2002).

More specifically, communitarianism provides a response to the liberal objection that public health interventions infringe on individual freedoms. This, says the communitarian, is just another specific ramification of the liberal's exaggerated and incoherent emphasis on atomistic individuals and their right to freely pursue their choices. In other words, public health in general, and specific public health initiatives, are bound to be perceived with hostility in a political culture that distortingly emphasizes individuals and their liberties, at the expense of a proper regard for communities and communal values. The liberal objection is an expression of this hostility. It can and should be corrected for; communitarianism is an academic contribution to this corrective exercise.

Three problems with the appeal to communitarianism in public health ethics

So far, then, communitarianism seems like a compelling counter to the liberal objection to public health. However, is it as convincing as first appears? There are three main problems. The first is that 'communitarianism' does not refer to a single, coherent, unified political theory. On the contrary, numerous theories attract the communitarian label. Worse still, they vary considerably; even worse still, the varieties on offer cross-cut the established political spectrum. In other words, left-leaning and right-leaning communitarian political philosophies have emerged from the communitarian critique of liberal individualism. Some of them – notably the political communitarianism associated with Amitai Etzioni (1993) – have attracted sustained criticism from all liberal-minded commentators. In this regard, there is an important distinction between theories that are termed philosophical communitarianism and those termed political communitarianism (Bell 2012). The former centres on rather abstract disputes with liberals about things like competing conceptions of the self; the latter is more of a political movement that implements various strategies to try to influence the political agenda (Parker 1996; Swift 2001: 133–6). Also, whilst all communitarians think the atomistic view of people is mistaken, some endorse further appeals to human nature that are contentious even amongst communitarian thinkers:

> The communitarian view implicitly or explicitly implies a moral appeal
> to human nature, notably to the idea of a natural life span in the course
> of which some basic common ('natural') human goals can be achieved
> [i.e.] that there are certain basic moral goals in life, to be realized in the
> course of a natural life span, and whose realization is to be supported
> by society at large. (Zwart 1999: 33)

Another good example of how complex and confusing communitarian political philosophy is, distinguishes relativistic and universalistic versions (Swift 2001: 133–6). Relativistic communitarians think that different communities subscribe to different norms, and there is no way of adjudicating between sets of norms that clash; by contrast, universalistic communitarians 'believe in a single true form of the good society and its associated virtues' (Roberts and Reich 2002: 1057). The upshot is that the communitarian critique of liberal individualism supports quite diverse political positions at different points on the political spectrum (Heginbotham 1999).

So, the first thing that compromises the appeal to communitarianism in public health ethics is that 'communitarianism' is an umbrella term under which sits a rather mixed bag of theories. The second problem is related to this. A strong theme in the relevant literature focuses on whether, once the various versions of communitarianism have been properly delineated, there is really quite as much at stake between liberals and communitarians as at first appeared. Swift (2001: 136–62) is very good on this. He distinguishes seven objections to liberalism in the name of community, showing that each is, arguably, based on an inadequate account of liberalism. He suggests that, on more charitable accounts of liberalism, liberals are able to accommodate much of what communitarians want to say. Also relevant here is the tendency for one side or other in the debate to give the impression that there is more at stake than is really the case, by presenting a caricature of their opponent and then knocking down a 'straw man'. To give an example from the public health literature, Childress and Bernheim (2003) and Parmet (2003) criticize Gostin's (2003) tendency to define liberalism as a much more extreme and rather implausible version of libertarianism. In a similar vein, there is a literature on whether the debate is 'misconceived'. The main thought here is that, on the one hand, extreme versions of these two '-isms' are clearly at loggerheads, but tend to be unconvincing; on the other hand, the more plausible versions of liberalism and communitarianism tend to collapse into one another at various points (Caney 1992).

These two points – that there is not a single, coherent, unified communitarian theory, and that there might be less at stake between communitarians and liberals than at first appears – compromise the appeal to communitarianism in response to the liberal objection. And there is a further, more general problem: there is a danger that appeals to communitarianism merely re-describe, rather than resolve, the basic dilemma at the heart of public health ethics. The dilemma, established in the Introduction, is between individual rights to personal freedom, and communal benefit in the form of population health protection and gain. Liberal political philosophy supports the former, not least in the form of the liberal objection. Communitarianism underpins the latter, by critiquing liberalism and calling for a return to community. But this sounds suspiciously like the same trade-off – between the rights of the individual and the population perspective – in terms of political philosophy. If so, the liberal who prioritizes individual rights over communal benefit will respond to the appeal to communitarianism by simply resisting the appeal to community and the anti-liberal political philosophy on which it is based. (We return to this 're-description problem' in the Concluding Remarks at the end of this book.)

It would appear, then, that the appeal in public health ethics to the communitarian critique of liberalism is seriously compromised. At this point, one might simply give up on it. But this would be too quick. The facts that communitarianism is a mixed bag of theories, that liberals and communitarians can agree at some points, and that the liberal can simply dig in their heels do not mean there is nothing at stake in the liberalism–communitarianism debate. The debate captures and expresses an important clash of attitudes, from the more individualistic- to the community-minded, as described by the continuum outlined at the start of this section. So, whatever the philosophical niceties, we should not lose sight of the fact that the debate keys into an issue that is important in general, and to public health in particular. Even Swift, for all his deflationary arguments, suggests: 'Communitarian writings … have raised deep and crucial issues that remain central to the philosophical agenda' (p. 136). Furthermore, as mentioned above, many of the most influential contemporary public health ethicists think that the communitarian critique of liberal individualism can do some work in specific public health ethics debates. At the very least, communitarian ideas and values can help us to avoid naïvely assuming that liberalism and individualism are sacrosanct political doctrines. Communitarianism provides a political-philosophical discourse in which to couch support for public health interventions that prioritize communal over individual goods. So, the communitarian critique of liberal individualism should be allowed to inform public health ethics issues in whatever ways naturally arise. Hence, in subsequent chapters, the liberalism–communitarianism debate will be referred to at numerous points in discussions of substantive public health problems.

Concluding remarks

This chapter has focused on two rejoinders to the liberal objection that public health activities infringe on personal freedoms. In different ways, both take us beyond traditional liberalism. The first is libertarian paternalism, or 'nudge', which attempts to combine the libertarian insistence on personal freedom with paternalistic interventions. It was argued that, although a libertarian has legitimate theoretical objections to the nudge agenda, it can have a role in public health. However, some recently suggested applications were criticized to present general constraints on public health nudges. The second took us outside the liberal framework altogether: liberty-limiting public health policies might be justified by emphasizing the ideas and values of a non-liberal political theory, namely, communitarianism. Although concerns about communitarianism were discussed, it provides an important perspective on public health interventions, so will be invoked in subsequent chapters.

Part I Summary

We are now in a position to sum up the discussion in Part I. The moral basis of public health is utilitarianism. This invites the naïve view that any public health intervention is morally justified on the grounds that it promotes and protects the target population's health. But we have now encountered numerous rejoinders to such naïvety, of various kinds. There are rejoinders from within moral philosophy, including both consequentialist and non-consequentialist rejoinders (Chapters 1 and 2); and there is an important rejoinder from political philosophy, namely, the liberal objection, which was critiqued from both within and beyond traditional liberalism (Chapters 3 and 4).

There is an understandable reaction to the plethora of theoretical considerations discussed in Part I. It might seem natural to infer from these first four chapters that almost any view on the ethics of a public health intervention can be justified by some theory or other. In other words, since proponents of a public health intervention can appeal to one theory to back up their view, whilst opponents can appeal to a different theoretical perspective, referring to moral and political philosophy will not aid progress. But this is to misunderstand the role of moral and political theory in public health ethics. To hold a view on a public health intervention, then search for a piece of moral or political philosophy to back it up, is to get things the wrong way round. Rather, the idea is to understand the kinds of theoretical considerations relevant to public health ethics, then let that understanding inform deliberation. With this in mind, we turn in Part II to the ethics of some of the most important kinds of public health activity.

Part II Public Health Activities

Introduction to Part II

Part I has put in place theoretical perspectives on public health gained from moral and political philosophy. Part II moves on to discuss the ethics of specific kinds of public health activity. The theory explained in Part I will be drawn on as and when it is pertinent. An overview of the main arguments presented in Part II is provided in this Introduction.

It is natural to start Part II with epidemiology because this is the scientific basis of all public health intervention. The key to the discussion of epidemiology in Chapter 5 is to distinguish two sources of disquiet. First, there are philosophical concerns about the status or value of epidemiologic data. Specifically, three theoretical challenges to epidemiology are presented and discussed, and the theme common to them all is clarified. Second, there are ethical concerns of a more direct kind about actual epidemiologic research practices and activities. Distinctive features of epidemiological research programmes create distinctive ethical tensions; for example, what notion of consent is appropriate to the kind of large-scale data set analysis typical of epidemiology? And certain branches of, or subspecialties within, epidemiology, such as genetic epidemiology, present ethical challenges. Having discussed such issues in epidemiological ethics, Chapter 5 ends by invoking virtue ethics, one of the moral theories explained in Part I.

The main theme of Chapter 6 is another fundamental feature of public health, namely, the nature of health. What is health? Any suspicion that this is not an important topic for public health ethics is dispelled at the start of Chapter 6. Then two conceptual claims about the nature of health are presented. The first conceptual claim is that 'health' is an ambiguous notion. In other words, we are in a dilemma about the nature of health because there are two equally plausible and important conceptions of health, namely, the positive and negative conceptions. The second conceptual claim is that health is an evaluative concept on both the positive and negative conceptions. In other words, whether one is thinking of health negatively or positively, one has in mind a value-laden notion and state. The rest of Chapter 6 explains the practical impact of these conceptual claims. First, the general impact on public health practice is explained. Then the importance of the ambiguous nature of health for health promotion is discussed. Finally, problems for other kinds of public health activity that emanate from the facts that health is ambiguous and value-laden are described.

Health promotion emerges from the discussion of the nature of health in Chapter 6 as a major theme. Chapter 7 pursues this by exploring the ethics of, arguably, the most interesting and contentious form of health promotion, namely, behaviour modification. The chapter begins by clarifying health promotion as behaviour modification. This generates two worries that are presented and discussed. The first worry is that behaviour modification smacks of victim-blaming; the second is that interventions to modify health behaviours are always and inevitably epistemically insecure. This is followed by a sketch of the principal means by which health promoters try to modify behaviours, and the ethical issues raised by them. The last section of Chapter 7 outlines the main ways of justifying interventions intended to change health behaviours. This involves unpacking the important concept of empowerment, and discussing whether and how coercing people to change their health behaviours can be justified.

Like Chapter 7, the focus of Chapter 8 is health behaviour. But whereas Chapter 7 discussed techniques for changing people's behaviour, the discussion is Chapter 8 centres on harm reduction, i.e., policies which aim not at eradicating but at ameliorating the harmful effects of risky behaviour. After discussing the definition of harm reduction we turn to the ethics of the approach. The discussion is structured by two distinctions. First, two research questions are distinguished: whether harm reduction in general is justified, and whether specific harm reduction policies are justified. It is argued that the latter is the more pressing research question. The second distinction is between harm reduction interventions aimed at legal versus illicit behaviour. Theoretical perspectives introduced in Part I are applied to both. The rest of Chapter 8 discusses the ethics of some particularly interesting and controversial harm reduction strategies.

Chapter 9 focuses on immunization, a major form of primary prevention. The central dilemma in vaccination ethics – between allowing vaccinees to choose to opt out of mass immunization programmes and coercing them to participate – is explained. Two perspectives on this dilemma – that of the State and that of the individual – are distinguished. Then, three lines of argument are pursued. First, is compulsory participation justified by appeal to the harm principle? Second, does a strong general duty not to infect others justify compulsory participation? And third, can the general proscription against free-riding be invoked in this context? The drift of the arguments in Chapter 9 is towards scepticism about the State coercing people to get vaccinated, centrally because mass immunization programmes are complex affairs that merit principled dissension.

Screening is an important form of secondary prevention. Chapter 10 explains and discusses the ethics of screening. The chapter is in three parts. The first describes the nature of screening, and current and proposed screening programmes. The middle section of the chapter looks at generic issues, i.e., ethical worries and criteria that apply to any screening programme. The third and final part of the chapter analyses one important facet of screening ethics by exploring the theme of benefit. Two slippery slopes are discerned: towards screening that is not to the benefit of true positives; and towards screening for the sake of non-medical benefits. Regarding the first slippery slope, the Kantian argument that some antenatal screening programmes turn true positives into mere means, as opposed to ends-in-themselves, is presented and discussed. Regarding the second slippery slope, screening for information is taken as a case study; three kinds of health information for which we can screen are juxtaposed.

5 Epidemiology |

The aim of this chapter is to provide a route through the substantial and expanding body of literature on epidemiology. The key to mapping this area is to distinguish two kinds of issues. First, there are theoretical or philosophical problems about the science of epidemiology. These are very fundamental challenges – problems with epidemiology in principle as opposed to epidemiology in practice – that bring into question the nature of the whole enterprise. Such problems are dealt with first because, if they are well founded, epidemiology, and the public health endeavours based on it, would be severely compromised. They are explained in the first section of this chapter, where some ways of meeting them are suggested, under the subheadings of frameworks, causation, and underdetermination and incommensurability. The second set of issues comprises problems for epidemiology in practice. There is a further distinction to be made here. On the one hand, there are worries about epidemiological techniques, such as the insinuation of spurious methods and explanations of exposure–disease associations. These will not be discussed in this book because our focus is on philosophical and ethical themes as opposed to the technicalities of epidemiological analysis (Wing 1994: 76–80). On the other hand, there are ethical problems that arise in the actual practice of epidemiologic research; these are the subject of the second section of this chapter. The main kinds of ethical challenges presented by epidemiologic studies are distinguished and described. The chapter ends by invoking a moral theory introduced and explained in Part I, namely, virtue ethics. Virtue ethics is especially useful in this context because the challenges to epidemiology discussed in the first two sections imply certain virtues.

Theoretical challenges to epidemiology

Epidemiology provides public health's scientific foundations. The science of epidemiology has two main, interrelated aims: the empirical study of the distribution and determinants of diseases in human populations, and the application of findings from such studies to control diseases and improve health. Epidemiologists also provide related data concerning, for example, the distribution of, and access to, health resources. Assessments about the health characteristics of a population, the distribution and causes of diseases in that population, and recommendations for interventions to protect and promote the population's health, are made on the basis of epidemiologic evidence. So, the validity of public health depends in no small part on the validity of epidemiology (Krieger 1994: 888; Rothman and Greenland 1998; Rothman 2002).

This section discusses objections to epidemiology in principle, i.e., theoretical or philosophical challenges that raise the concern that epidemiology does not report the kind of secure, scientific, objective knowledge about diseases on which public health interventions ought to be based. Three theoretical challenges are considered. The first centres on the fact that epidemiologists work within diverse theoretical frameworks (Krieger and Zierler 1996). The second focuses on epidemiologists' use of the concept of causation when making claims such as 'smoking causes lung cancer' (Parascandola and Weed 2001). The third applies the concepts of underdetermination and incommensurability from the philosophy of science to epidemiology (Weed 1997). At the end of the section, the common root shared by these three objections is uncovered.

Frameworks

First, as Krieger and Zierler (1996) point out, epidemiologists work within theoretical frameworks or epidemiologic theory (these terms are used interchangeably). They cite 'biomedical, lifestyle, cultural, behavioral, and social production of disease' (p. 107) as examples of such frameworks, and contrast these epidemiologic theories with two other main types of theories called for in epidemiology, namely, theories of causation and of error (we look at the problem emanating from causation in the next subsection). Krieger and Zierler's point is that a researcher's choice of framework influences their studies. As they put it, in epidemiology, frameworks in large part determine 'what we know, what we consider knowable, and what we ignore' (p. 109). Consequently, researchers working on the same disease within different frameworks will look at the disease differently, reach different conclusions about it and, in turn, recommend different public health responses.

Krieger and Zierler illustrate the point by reference to two theories, namely, lifestyle and social production of disease. They consider each of these as 'frameworks for generating hypotheses regarding the single question: what explains the distribution of [HIV/AIDS]?' (p. 108). It will be worth quoting their illustrative material quite fully:

> the interconnected explanatory ideas named as lifestyle theory posit: (1) individuals choose ways of living that have health consequences; (2) what epidemiologists measure on a population level are aggregates of these individual choices; and (3) individualized interventions can alter the distribution of these choices, and ultimately, of disease [...] Investigators base their study hypotheses, designs, and interpretations on these assumptions. For example, research premised on a lifestyle framework focuses on inadequate use of condoms (and of sterile needles) as the principal explanation for patterns of HIV incidence within and across different geographical regions. (P. 108)

Lifestyle theory, the first of Krieger and Zierler's illustrative frameworks, is then contrasted with another, namely, social production of disease theories that,

> provide interconnected explanatory ideas that posit: (1) the relative social and economic positioning of people shapes their exposures, including behaviors; (2) what epidemiologists measure on a population level are attributes of this positioning; and (3) population level interventions shift structural conditions that cause material and social deprivation, and thus alter societal distribution of disease. Hypotheses emerging from this theory propose explanations of HIV transmission in relation to: social class, access to health related resources, work place conditions, and discrimination. (P. 108)

In sum, epidemiology is framed by theories such as lifestyle and social production; change the framework, and the epidemiology of the same disease changes.

Krieger and Zierler do not themselves claim to have found an insurmountable theoretical objection to epidemiology. Rather, their aim is to advocate a more self-aware epidemiology, in the sense that epidemiologists recognize the variety of frameworks for, and their influence on, epidemiological studies and, consequently, take seriously the need for epidemiologic theory (we return to these ideas in the last section of this chapter, when the virtue of self-awareness in this context is discussed). But the way Krieger and Zierler juxtapose frameworks surely lends itself to the suggestion that epidemiology is in trouble because frameworks influence studies and there is a plethora of frameworks for epidemiologists to choose from. It could easily be taken to imply that, since epidemiologists working within different frameworks reach different conclusions, the result is a hotchpotch of perspective-driven views rather than linear progress in the science of diseases. This, in turn, threatens to undermine our confidence in ensuing public health recommendations.

How might such a frameworks problem be met? It would be a bad idea to question the phenomenon Krieger and Zierler describe because it seems evident that the same disease is studied in different ways by researchers who adopt different theoretical orientations. Nonetheless, the obvious thought elicited by Krieger and Zierler's examples is, why not do both: in other words – and referring back to the two theories described in the quotes above – why not take the perspective provided by both the lifestyle and social production of disease frameworks, and synthesize the results? After all, HIV is a very complex disease, a multi-faceted phenomenon, and both behaviours and socio-economic positioning are relevant to our understanding of it. In fact, lots of other features are important too, including sexual politics, addiction theory, political structures and biochemical mechanisms. A single framework was never going to be sufficient to 'capture' such a disease. Given this, far from being problematic, the only responsible kind of epidemiology of HIV involves numerous studies from within different frameworks. Some people will look at behavioural factors, others at social structures, and so on. Otherwise, epidemiologists are failing to do justice to the complexity of the disease in question.

There are worries about this rejoinder to the frameworks problem. Practical problems with looking at diseases from a variety of theoretical perspectives might arise. For example, some frameworks may not be adopted because of insufficient funds or the unwarranted pre-eminence of one framework over worthy alternatives. But these are not deep, theoretical problems with the science of epidemiology, and they are (in principle, at least) resolvable. What is perhaps more worrying is that the inclusive approach recommended here requires a second level of analysis: diverse epidemiologic data about, say, HIV acquired by epidemiologists working within different frameworks have to be synthesized in order to build up the complex picture this complex disease requires. And, it could be argued, data acquired from within different frameworks cannot be synthesized. Perhaps frameworks are incompatible in the sense that adopting one rules out others; or, although a disease can be studied from within different epidemiologic theories, the conclusions and recommendations about that disease emanating from different theoretical perspectives are mutually incompatible.

But is there really any reason to be so pessimistic? Recalling Krieger and Zierler's examples, arguably, there is no reason to think that studying HIV and behaviour is incompatible with studying socio-economic positioning and HIV, or that interventions recommended by the conclusions reached in one study contradict those reached in the other. Support for this view is discernible in Krieger and Zierler's text: it is implied by the mention of 'behaviors' in their depiction of social production of disease theories, which suggests that, far from being incompatible, there is cross-over between the two frameworks they discuss. This implies that, though there might seem to be a deep theoretical difficulty about epidemiology – namely, that research is framed by diverse epidemiologic theories – arguably, this is not a problem so much as a requirement on epidemiology given the multi-faceted nature of its subject matter. Investigations of, say, HIV should be undertaken from within diverse frameworks, the results being synthesized to build up a multi-faceted picture of the disease. There can be practical difficulties in achieving this, but no deep theoretical difficulty.

Causation

The second kind of theoretical challenge to epidemiology centres on the concept of causation. To introduce this, recall that the aim of epidemiology is to explain – in order to address – diseases in human populations. The obvious way to explain a disease is to discover and report its cause. Hence, aetiology, the study of the causes of diseases, is the major part of epidemiology, public health interventions being recommended to combat diseases by addressing their causes. In order to arrive at such causal claims one has to be able to distinguish causes from associations (Hill 1965; Susser 1991; for a brief survey of the historical development of causal inference in epidemiology, see Weed 1997: 113–14). In other words, lots of events are associated with diseases, but we are not interested in them because, since they do not cause the disease, addressing them would not combat it. Also, various factors can deflect epidemiologists from uncovering causes of disease, such as systematic and random errors, confounding variables, and bias (Brennan and Croft 1994). So, in order to succeed, epidemiologists need to factor these out of their analyses. The point is that it is the causes that epidemiologists are after, so causation (or causality) is central to epidemiology.

What is the problem? One way to explain it is to say that there would not be a problem if we knew what a cause is, i.e., if we understood the nature of causation. But causality is a very problematic notion. The place to look for theories of causation is metaphysics, a branch of philosophy. Metaphysicians are interested in the nature of reality or the world, specifically, in aspects of reality not amenable to natural sciences such as physics (hence, '*meta*physics'). Lots of things happen in the world (for convenience, let's call all these 'events'), some events are in causal relationships, so metaphysicians are interested in the nature of causation. But the question as to what a cause is has proved inordinately difficult to answer. We do not need to go further into philosophical details to get the general point that 'there is no single, clearly articulated definition [of the concept of causation]' (Parascandola and Weed 2001: 905; see also Weed and Gorelic 1996).

Left at this, there still might not seem to be much of a problem. After all, there is 'no single, clearly articulated definition' of 'friendship', for example, either, but when someone says, 'he is my friend', we know roughly what is meant and can proceed with the conversation. Likewise, we know roughly what 'smoking causes lung cancer' on cigarette packets is meant to say. But, as Parascandola and Weed point out,

> despite much discussion of causes, it is not clear that epidemiologists are referring to a single shared concept.
>   Multiple definitions of cause have been offered in epidemiology [...]
> In practice, many causal statements are ambiguously stated; for example, 'smoking is a cause of cancer' may mean 'every smoker will develop cancer' or it can become construed as 'at least one smoker will develop cancer,' depending upon the underlying concept of causation the speaker has in mind. (2001: 905)

So, the problem is not so much a lack of clarity as ambiguity: a typical aetiological claim, such as that smoking is a cause of cancer, means different things depending on the speaker's understanding of causation. The analogy would be that people might mean quite different

things by 'he is my friend' depending on which of the competing definitions of friendship they have in mind; we could proceed with the
conversation, but might well be talking past one another.

In a very useful survey of epidemiologic literature, Parascandola
and Weed (2001) delineate five definitions of causation in use in contemporary epidemiology. The first is that 'C causes E' means C produces E, or C makes E happen. As Parascandola and Weed rightly
point out, this might be a way 'cause' is used in epidemiology, but it
is a hopeless understanding of causality because the only way of flesh-
ing out what 'produces' or 'makes happen' means here is to say something like, 'produces in the sense of causes'. So we end up with a
circular definition: 'cause' is defined in terms of 'produces', which is
defined in terms of 'causes'.

The next definition Parascandola and Weed delineate is based on
the idea that a cause is a necessary condition. A necessary condition
is a condition without which the effect cannot occur. According to this
second understanding of causation, 'C causes E' means that C is a
necessary condition for E. For example, one cannot have AIDS without
being HIV+, so HIV is a necessary condition for AIDS. On this
account, HIV causes AIDS. But this is an unconvincing definition. It
is true that some diseases are caused by necessary conditions. But we
are left with a very narrow account of disease causation. On this
account, a high cholesterol level is not a cause of heart disease, nor is
smoking a cause of lung cancer, because a high cholesterol level is not
a necessary condition for heart disease (one can have heart disease
despite a low cholesterol level), nor is smoking a cause of lung cancer
(one can have lung cancer despite being a non-smoker).

Their next definition involves 'sufficient-component causes'. A sufficient cause is a condition given which the effect must occur: 'C causes
E' means that, given C, E has to occur. The important variant on this
is where there are lots of conditions, no one of which is sufficient for
an effect, but which, taken together, form a complex sufficient condition for that effect. (This is the basis of the philosophical account of
causation in Mill (1950) and Mackie (1974), famously adapted by
Rothman (1976) to epidemiology.) So, for example, exposure to the
measles virus is not sufficient to develop measles (you could be exposed
to the virus but not get measles). But exposure to the measles virus is
a necessary component; it combines with a number of other conditions
to form a complex sufficient cause of measles. So, 'C causes E' means
that C is one of a number of conditions (a 'component') which, altogether, are sufficient for E to occur.

The last two definitions of causation Parascandola and Weed discern in the literature invoke probabilistic causes and counter-factual causes. According to probabilistic causation, 'C causes E' means that C makes it more likely that E will occur. According to counter-factual causation, 'C causes E' means that, had C not obtained, E would not have occurred or would have been less likely to occur. Parascandola and Weed suggest that the best definition of causation (at least, for epidemiology) combines these two, the probabilistic and the counter-factual. So, their suggestion is that 'smoking causes lung cancer' means: if you do smoke you are more likely to – and if you do not smoke, you are less likely to – get lung cancer. In arguing for this definition, they suggest that it can incorporate the insights of alternatives. Furthermore, Parascandola and Weed ask why commentators resist their account (p. 909). Here they refer to two controversies in epidemiology which, they suggest, impact on one's preference for one or other definition of causation:

(a) Causal explanations of diseases take place at different levels. For example, a biochemical explanation of lung cancer takes place at a lower level than does social explanations of smoking patterns. Some people think that the only real causal explanations are micro-level ones, because this is proper science. Others think that there is no hierarchy here, and that data from various levels of analysis can be relevant to diseases.

(b) Epidemiology has a split focus between doing science and making public health recommendations. Some people think, first and foremost, epidemiologists are scientists interested in the objective truth about their subject-matter; i.e., they aim to provide accurate and objective scientific facts about diseases. Others demur, suggesting that the point of epidemiology is to provide underpinnings for public health policy. Sometimes, epidemiologists do both. (See Greenland 1988; Susser 1991; Weed and Gorelic 1996; we return to this dispute in the next section)

Parascandola and Weed get two things absolutely right. First, they argue for an inclusive theory of causation (recall that their definition of causation combines the probabilistic and the counter-factual). In other words, rather than claiming that their preferred notion of causation is correct, and simply dismissing alternatives, they show how it includes the good things about its alternatives. For example, they point out that their definition allows for necessary and sufficient causes, and accommodates determining causes. The second thing they get right is that apparently diverse views in this area actually map on to one another. In other words, certain views go hand-in-hand. For example, if you think the real causes of diseases are to be found at the micro-level of biological mechanisms, then you will think of cause deterministically not probabilistically; and if you think the aim of epidemiology is scientific truth (public health recommendations being a by-product) then you will be sympathetic to both these views.

These two ideas from Parascandola and Weed are crucial to defusing the theoretical challenge to epidemiology that is based on the notion of causation: first, we need an account of causation in epidemiology that is broad, in the sense that it does not rule out anything that might be important in combating diseases; and second, we need to appreciate how apparently diverse views go hand-in-hand. But, although this is very much in the spirit of Parascandola and Weed's article, one thing about their position is disconcerting. For all their insight into the need for inclusiveness and combinations of views, in the end they do opt for a specific definition of causation: 'We argue that the probabilistic definition combined with a counter-factual condition ... provides the greatest promise for epidemiology' (p. 909). So, they are still playing the game of defining causation. And this is a dangerous game because it makes epidemiology dependent on success in metaphysics. Suppose someone were to present a convincing counter-example or counter-argument to Parascandola and Weed's suggested account of causality. Then we would be back to the drawing board, epidemiology being put on hold until someone patches up the metaphysics, lest epidemiologists start talking past each other again.

So, perhaps we should adopt the spirit of Parascandola and Weed's suggestion, but push it a bit further. We do not need to define 'causation' – or provide a general causal theory – at all. What we do need is to recognize a continuum between two positions, viewpoints or perspectives. Each pole of the continuum includes different but closely related sets of views. The first pole can be roughly labelled 'scientific'. At this end of the continuum, people think quite postivistically about diseases. Epidemiologists study diseases in the spirit in which chemists study chemicals. The aim of epidemiology is scientific truth. This means looking at the micro-level of molecules and doing biochemistry in order to discover and report the (typically singular) cause of a disease. They focus on factors that determine that a disease will develop. The opposite end of the continuum can be roughly labelled 'public health'. Here, people think that epidemiology is not an end in itself but a means to combating disease. So, whilst the biochemistry is important, the aim is to explain or understand the disease phenomenon in broader than merely positivistic terms. This allows for explanations of health and disease that are made up of societal and behavioural, as well as natural-scientific, strands. Factors that only make a disease more likely to occur are relevant; in fact, if these are the only ones we can do anything about, they become the most relevant factors.

The continuum just outlined can be summarized as shown in Table 5.1.

So, what presented itself as a very complicated picture, including lots of definitions of causation, ambiguity and various underpinning controversies, has resolved itself into a pretty straightforward continuum between two epidemiologic perspectives. Now the question is, how threatening is this continuum to the business of epidemiology?

It is hard to see any major theoretical objection to epidemiology here. Both sets of views at the two poles of the continuum are coherent, and both are important: to combat AIDS, for example, we need to know about both the biomechanics of HIV and the habits of intravenous drug users (for a different, neat example see Renton 1994: 82–3). Since the overall aim is to recommend interventions, different kinds of information will be important at different times. It depends on the context, notably on whether there is a way of disrupting molecular-level mechanisms or macro-level social and behavioural processes. So, different places on the continuum will be appropriate depending on the nature of the disease in question and the opportunities for effective interventions. No part of the continuum is just plain wrong for epidemiology, though, of course, at any one point in time epidemiology can be at the wrong place on the continuum given the nature of the disease

Table 5.1 The science–public health continuum

Scientific	Public health
The aim of epidemiology is to report scientific facts; causes of diseases are found at the micro-level (especially, in biological process); diseases have a single cause; diseases have determining causes.	The aim of epidemiology is to recommend public health interventions; causes of diseases are found at the macro-level (including behavioural and social factors); diseases have multiple causes ('webs of causation'); diseases have probabilistic causes.

under investigation (cf. Rothman 1988; Krieger 1994; Susser and Susser 1996a, 1996b). The spirit of the response to the theoretical threat to epidemiology from the nature of causation recommended in this section is nicely summed up by Weed (1996: 82):

> a theory of breast cancer occurrence ... must incorporate not only biology and lifestyle risk factors, but also ... social structures and the like. Given the current status of theory development in epidemiology, this seems a difficult and distant task.
>
> Nevertheless, theoretical development in epidemiology should be encouraged ...

Underdetermination and incommensurability

The third kind of theoretical challenge to epidemiology centres on the concepts of underdetermination and incommensurability. The key to this is to distinguish and clarify these rather intimidating concepts. 'Underdetermination' refers to the fact that the evidence underdetermines theories or hypotheses:

> Epidemiologists and other practitioners of causal influence already are familiar with underdetermination, if not by name then in concept. (The term 'uncertainty' is more likely to be used.) Epidemiologic evidence, comprised of (often loosely) summarized estimates of effect in population-based studies, *underdetermines* the hypotheses that can explain that evidence. (Weed 1997: 112)

To illustrate, consider a typical epidemiological claim, such as, 'induced abortions cause breast cancer'. The claim is a hypothesis, or theory. There are alternative hypotheses (most notably that induced abortions do not cause breast cancer). Epidemiologists acquire and analyse evidence, in the form of epidemiologic data, to determine which is true. Ideally, the evidence would establish (prove or 'determine') the truth of the correct hypothesis. But it does not. Rather, hypotheses are 'underdetermined' in the sense that we cannot adjudicate between competing hypotheses just by looking to the evidence. Roughly, various hypotheses are supportable by the evidence (McMullin 1995).

Given underdetermination, the incommensurability problem follows (Veatch and Stempsey 1995). How are epidemiologists to proceed if they cannot rely on the evidence to prove or disprove their hypotheses? They evaluate the relevant evidence by reference to their value system. Such values can be more or less explicit. There are scientific values 'such as empirical accuracy, consistency, fertility, simplicity, and the like' (Weed 1997: 111). There are also 'extrascientific values, such as moral positions, cultural norms, and political ideologies, that are relevant to the evidence and its assessment' (Weed 1997: 111). 'Wish bias' – roughly, the influence of the fact that the researcher already believes their hypothesis to be true – has been highlighted as an especially important extrascientific value in epidemiology (Wynder et al. 1990; Weed and Kramer 1996). Different scientists have different value systems. 'Incommensurability' refers to the fact that scientists' value systems can be different in the sense that there is no convincing way of adjudicating between them, because there is no independent way of deciding who has the 'right' values. This problem can be more or less severe. If scientists approach data using completely different values, the incommensurability is total; partial incommensurability results when value systems are significantly, but not wholly, different. The upshot is that quite different epidemiological claims can be supported by the same body of epidemiological evidence. (For an indicative list of 'sources of incommensurability', see Weed 1997: 116–18.)

Underdetermination and incommensurability are topics in the philosophy of science, and there is not time to get too deeply into these here. Nonetheless, some lines of thought can be introduced by way of a response. One rejoinder is to question whether the problem is really as dramatic as all that. Of course, scientific and extrascientific values can influence scientific research, but is there any reason to think this is more than an occasional and relatively benign problem in epidemiology? Weed (1997) suggests there is. For one thing, he points out that the problem, and appreciation of it by epidemiologists, seems to be on the increase. Perhaps even more tellingly, he suggests why this might be so. Specifically, 'the relatively brief formal exposure to causal inference methodology [in, e.g., epidemiologic training] coupled with a practice that permits a considerable individualized approach [results in] a situation in which differences in scientific values can emerge and even flourish' (p. 120).

So, we need a better rejoinder than merely dismissing the problem. Here are two suggestions. The underdetermination–incommensurability problem gets going because of a certain picture of scientific enquiry: science is a neutral method for discovering objective facts about the world. Given this picture, the revelation that scientific 'findings' are 'contaminated' by such things as enquirers' values is devastating. Science comes to seem fundamentally flawed. But the revelation is devastating only because of the original picture of science. Perhaps that picture was always very unrealistic; given a more appropriate depiction of the scientific enterprise, the value-laden nature of science would not seem so threatening.

Two alternative ways of depicting science are as follows. To introduce the first, consider a comment by Wing (1994: 83):

> Belief that truth is something which is found 'out there' rather than something that is made from observations of the world using socially and culturally produced languages and concepts is partly a reaction to the mistaken perception that the only alternative to value-free scientific objectivity is relativism and the abandonment of any basis for making comparative evaluations of scientific explanations. But recognition that all knowledge, including scientific knowledge, is rooted in social constructs does not negate the idea of objectivity in the sense of fairness, justice, and intellectual honesty.

The idea is this. Lurking behind the underdetermination–incommensurability problem is the assumption that science is meant to be objective, the value-laden is not objective (or, conversely, only the value-neutral is objective), science is value-laden, therefore science is not objective. But what is meant by 'objective' should be a matter of debate, not simply assumed. As Wing points out, no method of enquiry – science or any other – is entirely neutral in all respects. This should alert us to the possibility that objectivity (objective truth or knowledge) is achieved by acquiring and interpreting data by reference to a set of values. In which case, the fact that scientists bring their values to bear on their work might not debar them from presenting objective facts.

This attempt to divorce objectivity and value-neutrality will not sound convincing to someone who insists that the evaluative is subjective. So, here is another tack. One might accentuate the pragmatic over the epistemological value of science. In other words, perhaps it is more important to stress the fact that science enables us to do things, rather than that science gives us knowledge or truths about the world. Of course, science only enables us to do things because it provides us with knowledge; but, on this account of science, it is not the pursuit of knowledge, unadulterated by anything as 'subjective' as values, that is science's *raison d'être*. This move does not solve the underdetermination–incommensurability problem exactly, but it does ameliorate it: provided our science enables us to live better in the world, it is doing its job. The fact that theories are underdetermined and value-laden no longer seems like such a problem. (For other responses to the underdetermination–incommensurability problem, see Bayley 1995; Weed 1997: 112ff.)

Commonalities

So far, three theoretical challenges to epidemiology have been discussed. It is important to keep these apart because they are different from one another. Frameworks, causes and values are not synonymous so, in pursuing these problems, different considerations are relevant to them. Nonetheless, the three are obviously connected. To quote one example: 'Partial incommensurability exists within epidemiology ... Its presence and effects can be found in the practice of causal inference' (Weed 1997: 123). Furthermore, all three of the theoretical problems discussed here share the same root. In their different ways, all three are challenging the assumption that there are objective facts about diseases which epidemiologists dispassionately discover and report. The frameworks problem says that an epidemiologist's epidemiologic theory influences their work; the causation problem says that an epidemiologist's understanding of causality influences their work; and the incommensurability problem says that an epidemiologist's scientific and other values influence their work. In each case, the point is that epidemiology is not the neutral reporting of objective facts about diseases but, rather, an interpretative enterprise subject to a variety of influences. From this point the discussion could go in several directions. Staying with the theoretical, one might question whether data really are subject to interpretation in the ways these theoretical problems suggest, or draw parallels from discussions of similar worries about other sciences. But, since our focus is on ethics, let's move on to some of the now traditional ethical worries about epidemiology and return to these theoretical challenges at the end of this chapter.

Ethical issues in epidemiologic research

Background

Two kinds of issues about epidemiology were distinguished at the start of this chapter. The second kind comprises ethical challenges that arise during the actual practice of epidemiologic research. These are discussed in this section. An important part of the background to this is 'research ethics'. The development of research ethics has been motivated in large part by the clear recognition of the ongoing need for better research governance which grew out of infamous atrocities, including those perpetrated by Nazis during the Second World War, dubious trials such as the Tuskegee Syphilis Study, and more recent offences, such as the Alder Hey children's organs retrieval scandal in the United Kingdom.

The response has seen the clarification of the general ethical dilemma at the heart of research between the benefits to be gained from acquiring and applying data, on the one hand, and risks to and burdens on participants, on the other. This dilemma is more complicated than it sounds. For example, research can actually harm participants or, alternatively, put participants at risk of being harmed. Both these outcomes are concerning, and there is a requirement on the part of researchers to avoid them. Furthermore, there are different kinds of burdens. Some research creates actual physical or psychological harm, ranging from participants being inconvenienced and made anxious, to suffering discomfort and even pain. By contrast, some research creates moral wrongs, such as infringing participants' rights to privacy and self-determination. There are numerous grey areas in research ethics. For example, it sounds neat to contrast benefits and burdens, but this belies the way that medical research actually progresses. Very often it is not possible to ascertain whether a research programme will be useful, how beneficial it will prove to be. Many of the most beneficial medico-scientific advances have been achieved by research, the value of which was quite unanticipated. The fact that it is so difficult to predict accurately the benefits that accrue from research makes the trade-off between benefits and burdens very difficult.

The important point in this brief sketch is the increased awareness of the need for research governance, including a quite general demand that all research involving human participants is subject to ethical scrutiny. Epidemiology, which comprises a set of research activities involving human subjects, is not (or should not be) exempt. In addition, some specific features of epidemiologic research have motivated concerns about the ethics of epidemiologic studies. For one thing, ethical issues in epidemiology have been raised by new public health challenges, such as the public health response to the HIV pandemic. For another, new kinds of epidemiology that arise due to recent advances in medical science – for example, molecular epidemiology, based on new opportunities in genetic medicine – have forced ethics into the limelight. As a result, interest in epidemiological ethics has increased markedly. Conversely, the focus on ethics has helped clarify the nature of epidemiology (Coughlin and Beauchamp 1996b; Coughlin 2000).

Two interconnected developments in epidemiological ethics are worth stressing. First, on the academic front, two early landmark texts were published: the *Journal of Clinical Epidemiology, 44, Supplement*

1, was devoted to the ethics of epidemiology; and Coughlin and Beauchamp (1996a) edited a collection of papers on the same theme. Subsequently, numerous important contributions to the academic debate about the nature of, and appropriate responses to, ethical challenges in epidemiologic practice have been published (Coughlin 2006). Second – and in part due to these academic efforts – there has been the gradual integration of ethics into the profession of epidemiology. For example, there is an ongoing effort to ensconce ethics in standard epidemiologic curricula (Coughlin and Etheridge 1995; Goodman and Prineas 1996; Coughlin 1996a; Rossignol and Goodmonson 1995). It is now commonplace for ethics to be on the agenda of meetings of international epidemiologic organizations. And professional standards for epidemiologists (Last 1996; Coughlin 1996b) have been promoted in various ethics guidelines, codes of ethics and professional codes of conduct for epidemiologists (Last 1990; Sleep 1991; Weed and Coughlin 1999). Notable examples include the Ethics Guidelines of the American College of Epidemiology (American College of Epidemiology 2000; cf. McKeown 2000; McKeown et al. 2003); the International Epidemiological Association's European Federation's document, *Good Epidemiological Practice* (International Epidemiological Association's European Federation 2007); and the Council for International Organizations of Medical Sciences' *International Ethical Guidelines on Epidemiological Studies* (Council for International Organizations of Medical Sciences 2009).

Before developing a more detailed survey of epidemiological ethics, a point is worth emphasizing. One might think that the nature of epidemiology is such that really serious ethical issues do not arise: after all, epidemiologists tend to use large bodies of health information as their primary data source, so the opportunities for perpetrating really dramatic harms on human subjects are far fewer than in clinical trials:

> The risks posed by nonexperimental epidemiologic studies are often minor compared with those that must be considered in designing and conducting clinical trials and other experimental studies, and surveys of respondents' attitudes toward participation in epidemiologic studies have suggested that many subjects find the experience personally satisfying or rewarding. (Coughlin 1996c: 146)

It is true that there are types of research that raise more obvious and dramatic ethical problems than does epidemiology. One only has to think of animal experimentation, or cloning embryos for stem cell research, to see this. But, as Coughlin goes on from the previous quote to clarify, it would be a mistake to conclude that ethics is irrelevant to epidemiology. For one thing, some ethical concerns arise in all professional research activities (for example, duties and obligations around plagiarism and disseminating findings). So, ethics is important even to the conduct of epidemiologic studies that do not use human participants directly. And, as we shall see, epidemiologic research involving human participants raises some important and distinctive problems in its own right.

Consensus

Let's start with the numerous attempts to list issues familiar from generic research ethics (such as consent and confidentiality) that arise in epidemiology. A consensus seems to have developed on the dozen or so general obligations or duties incumbent on epidemiologists. A couple of examples should be enough to capture this consensus. In its ethics guidelines, the American College of Epidemiology (2000) lists epidemiologists' duties in terms of minimizing harms, maximizing benefits and justly distributing harms and benefits; protecting rights to confidentiality, privacy and informed consent; submitting studies for independent ethical review; maintaining trust and scientific standards; avoiding conflicts of interest; communicating ethical requirements within the discipline and confronting unethical research; properly reporting results and meeting various obligations to communities (including involving community representatives and respecting cultural diversity). Beauchamp (1996) contains a very similar list of responsibilities. Regarding participants, this includes welfare protection, informed consent, privacy, confidentiality, committee review; regarding society, it includes providing benefits, building trust, avoiding conflicts of interest, impartiality; regarding employers and funders, it includes formulating responsibilities, protecting privileged information; and, finally, regarding colleagues, it includes reporting methods and results, and reporting unacceptable conduct (cf. Beauchamp et al. 1991).

There is much more to say about each of these issues, but only time here to suggest a framework that might be useful for reflection. Two nexuses of ideas seem both prominent and very much connected. The first nexus is about risks and benefits. It is typical in epidemiological ethics to read that researchers are responsible for minimizing risks, maximizing benefits and ensuring that risks and benefits are judiciously balanced and distributed. But this begs the question as to the kinds of risks and benefits characteristic of epidemiology. Coughlin

(1996c) examines this in more detail, outlining the opportunities for risks and benefits typical in epidemiologic research programmes. Ultimately, the main kind of benefit epidemiology promises to deliver is public health gain: by explaining and describing the determinants and distribution of diseases, interventions to improve the public's health can be devised. Less straightforward is the main kind of harm epidemiology threatens to create. Here, Capron's (1991) distinction between harms and wrongs is important. Acknowledging that 'physical and psychological injuries' are unlikely to be caused by epidemiologic research, Capron explains that 'people may have been wronged even when they have not suffered harm'. Classic examples include 'invasion of your privacy without your consent'; another, which recalls Kant's ethics discussed in Chapter 2, involves treating people as means rather than ends-in-themselves (cf. Gold 1996: 131–3 who, like Capron, distinguishes individual and group harms).

This leads to the other main nexus of ideas typical of literature on epidemiological ethics. This includes notions such as consent, confidentiality and privacy. As Last (1996: 57) put it: 'The clash between the privacy rights of persons and the need for access to and disclosure of personal health-related information is the most frequent ethical dilemma to confront epidemiologists.' It is clear why this is so: to deny access to health-related information would entirely stifle epidemiology; but individual rights to disclose one's own health information is a basic tenet of research ethics. The connection between the two nexuses of ideas outlined here is that a principal source of moral concern in epidemiologic research is the transgression of the right to confidentiality and privacy, when epidemiologists make non-consented use of health-related information required for their studies (Capron 1991; Gold 1996; Bayer and Fairchild 2004: 476ff.).

Epidemiologic subspecialties and the advocacy issue

Apart from this consensus on the main generic issues in epidemiological ethics, challenges arise in specific branches, or sub-disciplines, of epidemiology. The point to note here is that, whilst all epidemiologists are interested in the distribution and determinants of disease in order to recommend interventions, epidemiology is very heterogeneous. There are various branches of this increasingly diverse discipline, including social, psychiatric, chronic disease, environmental, genetic and industrial epidemiology. These sub-disciplines take place within different research contexts. So, ethical challenges can arise that are distinctive to these different branches of epidemiology. A specific example will be enough to make the general point. Genetic epidemiology studies the interaction of genetic and environmental factors in diseases (Khoury et al. 1993; Holtzman and Andrews 1997; Thomas 2004). The important thing about genetic epidemiology is that it requires moving from the traditional epidemiological studies of unrelated participants to studying families. This creates distinctive ethical tensions. How does the familial nature of genetic epidemiology change the nature and type of consent required? What kinds of intra-familial consent are feasible? What kinds of threats to confidentiality arise here? How feasible is it that health-related information can remain discrete between family members? In some cases, the fact that distinctive ethical challenges can arise within epidemiological subfields has been well recognized, resulting in ethics guidelines specific to a subspecialty. For example, Soskolne and Light (1996) adapted generic ethics guidelines for epidemiology to produce ethics guidelines for environmental epidemiology.

There is one final issue that has already arisen but should be discussed a bit further. The basic question here is, are epidemiologists scientists, or do they have further social roles and responsibilities as public health advocates? This is a longstanding and ongoing dispute within epidemiology (Weed 1994; Weed and McKeown 2003). It can be traced back to the two aims of epidemiology distinguished at the start of this chapter, namely, the empirical study of diseases (which is the science facet), and the application of findings in the form of recommended public health interventions (the advocacy aspect). The upshot is 'considerable debate within the discipline about the extent to which epidemiologists as epidemiologists should be involved as advocates or policy makers in the practice of public health or should remain insulated from such activities in order to safeguard the objectivity of science' (McKeown et al. 2003: 210).

There are good arguments on both sides of this debate. For example, as the previous quote from McKeown et al. suggests, the 'scientists first' lobby can argue that, were epidemiologists to become public health advocates, objectivity might be compromised (cf. Krieger 1999). Also, it is dubious that epidemiologists are well prepared to play an advocacy role. On the other hand, policymaking can enhance scientific objectivity by motivating improvements in empirical methods (Weed and Mink 2002). And one might appeal to ethical theories to insist that epidemiologists have social responsibilities and an advocacy role. For example, Weed and McKeown analyse the concept of social responsibility, arguing that it would be incoherent for epidemiologists to be committed to public health as a social good, whilst eschewing responsibility for ensuring that their findings realize that social good. Weed (1994) appeals to the principle of beneficence (see Chapter 2), but suggests that whether an epidemiologist who advocates public health recommendations is merely justified in doing so – as opposed to being obligated to do so – largely depends on how the professional aims of epidemiology are described.

The reason this dispute is so entrenched is that there is not an obviously correct stance to take here. Because epidemiologists are scientists working in an area that has massive public health implications, their discipline has a dual aspect. This requires a sensible compromise. In other words, epidemiologists do not have a general duty to be advocates because, first and foremost, their job is to secure scientific data. Nonetheless, because of the nature of their discipline, circumstances can arise in which it would be remiss of an epidemiologist not to play a wider social role by undertaking advocacy. A simple example might be: findings that could provide significant public health benefits have, for whatever reason, not been fully appreciated, and the epidemiologist can either leave it at that and move on to their next research project, or take responsibility for publicizing and utilizing the data further. This avoids the 'scientist–advocate' stand-off. It also puts the onus on the epidemiologist to show good judgement and vision and implies that character and virtue are very relevant to the discipline, a point on which we can now expand.

Epidemiology and virtue ethics

There are various ways in which to address the themes discussed so far in this chapter. For example, a number of commentators have applied Beauchamp and Childress's four principles of biomedical ethics, which were discussed in Chapter 2, to ethical issues in epidemiologic research (Westrin et al. 1992; International Epidemiological Association's European Federation 2007). However, given the view expressed in Chapter 2 that these traditional biomedical principles apply poorly to public health ethics, a different approach is required. In this section, epidemiological ethics will be addressed via virtue ethics (Weed and McKeown 1998). This is because applying virtue ethics will enable us to bring together the two kinds of challenges to epidemiology discussed in this chapter, namely, the theoretical and the ethical.

To begin, let's recall from Chapter 2 that the main idea behind virtue ethics is to restore character and character traits to prominence in moral theory. So, in contrast to consequentialist theories (such as utilitarianism) which emphasize the outcome of actions, and to deontological theories (such as Kant's) which emphasize duties based on the nature (as opposed to the consequences) of actions, virtue ethics states that right action is that which results from the acquisition and exercise of the virtues. It seems clear that virtues are required to address the kinds of ethical problems surveyed in the previous section, i.e., ethical challenges presented by the practice of epidemiology. These problems require a sensitivity to such challenges and the right kind of character to deal with them. This is nicely summed up in the Ethics Guidelines of the American College of Epidemiology (American College of Epidemiology 2000: S3.1): 'Professional virtues are those traits of character that dispose us to act in ways that contribute to achieving the good that is internal to the practice of epidemiology.' The Guidelines cite an example: 'The time that senior epidemiologists spend mentoring graduate students and junior investigators in the proper design and conduct of epidemiologic studies.' The point is also made in the Guidelines that virtues are distinct from, though complementary to, duties, rules and obligations. So, the Guidelines make clear the extent to which the practice of epidemiology is enhanced by acquisition and exercise of the virtues (cf. Soskolne and MacFarlane 1996 on the opposite of professional virtue, namely, scientific misconduct).

What is not so obvious is that virtue ethics is also very relevant to the three theoretical challenges to epidemiology discussed in the first section of this chapter. Recall, these were the problems of frameworks, causation and underdetermination–incommensurability. Arguably, these three problems, and the rejoinders to them, imply certain virtues and, moreover, the kinds of virtues required are similar in all three cases. To introduce this, consider some comments by Barbor (1990) which, though specifically about alcohol epidemiology, apply more generally. Barbor is concerned by the fact that, '[d]espite their common interest in the basic purpose of epidemiology, the differences among alcohol epidemiologists are more apparent than the similarities' (p. 293). The 'differences' he has in mind are just the kinds of things captured by the theoretical objections to epidemiology discussed above – 'differences in opinion, belief and the interpretation of facts' (p. 293) – and the threat they present is that alcohol epidemiology will degenerate into 'a confusing panoply of conflicting methods, findings and conclusion' (p. 295). The important thing for our purposes is how Barbor recommends avoiding this threat, namely, through 'understanding these differences' (p. 293), and 'a better understanding of who [alcohol epidemiologists] are and what they are studying' (p. 295). In other words, Barbor puts the onus back on the epidemiologist to take responsibility for being of a certain professional character, i.e., someone prepared to understand the influences on their own and their colleagues' studies.

The point is that this implies virtue ethics. Consider, for example, a virtue such as self-awareness, captured in the idea that one is thoughtful and reflective about one's work, including being conscious of the wider context of one's studies and alternative ways of going about them. The corresponding vice is a bullish insistence on doing things in a preordained way, including insensitivity to, and reluctance to take on board the products of, alternative viewpoints. Roughly, the virtue is one of open-mindedness, the corresponding vice that of insularity. This virtue is implied by the rejoinders to all three theoretical problems discussed in the first section of this chapter.

First, epidemiologists work within frameworks. As was argued above, this need not be an insurmountable theoretical problem; but it will be unless epidemiologists take responsibility for being aware of their choice of frameworks, the availability of alternative frameworks and the need to synthesize findings achieved within different frameworks. Basically, it is incumbent on epidemiologists to be prepared to be explicit about the kind of epidemiology they are doing. For example, a study that addresses a disease by looking for behavioural factors needs to make clear that this is the researchers' preferred epidemiologic theory, and to make those findings available for synthesis with findings from within frameworks reasonably eschewed by the researchers.

Second, epidemiologists work with different conceptions of causality. Again, as argued above, this need not be an insurmountable theoretical problem; but it will be if certain virtues are lacking. It is incumbent on epidemiologists to understand and appreciate the 'science–public health' continuum outlined in the first section of this chapter because it is no good being so steeped in science, sociology, behaviour modification, or whatever, as to be blinkered to other kinds of explanations of diseases. The kind of epidemiology one does is defined by way of contrast with alternatives; in this case, by way of contrast with other positions on the continuum. Furthermore, epidemiologists should be prepared to move along the continuum as required by the demands of their research projects. This is particularly important. What is the point of doggedly pursuing, say, the micro-level causes of an incurable disease when behaviour modification can reduce prevalence and incidence rates? The right place to be on the continuum depends on the context; since the latter can change, epidemiologists must be sufficiently flexible and open-minded to occupy different places on the continuum.

The third theoretical problem discussed above centred on the paired concepts of underdetermination and incommensurability. This distilled down to the fact that epidemiology is influenced by (scientific and extrascientific) values, and value systems vary between researchers. Again, it was argued that this is not an insurmountable objection to the discipline. But, again, it will be unless virtues such as self-awareness are acquired and exercised. In this context, self-awareness means reflecting on the values one brings to the research, and the influence they have or might have on one's collection and interpretation of the data. It requires that epidemiologists are aware of, and receptive to, alternative values, including preparedness to change one's value system if this is what the study demands.

So, virtue ethics is relevant not only to the ethical challenges that arise in the practice of epidemiology described in the second part of this chapter: virtues (such as 'self-awareness') are also required if the theoretical problems discussed in the first part are not to prove insurmountable. Of course, there is much more to say, not least about the kinds of theoretical and ethical challenges epidemiology presents, the role of moral theories other than virtue ethics in meeting them, and, indeed, about the other virtues relevant to epidemiology. Nonetheless, enough has been said to endorse Weed and McKeown's suggestion:

> We hope to make a strong enough case for the relevance and importance of virtue ethics to warrant a claim that it is relevant to all ethical issues in epidemiology and so emerges as a necessary consideration in the epidemiologist's professional life. (1998: 343)

Concluding remarks

This chapter has explained the two main points of discussion about the ethics of epidemiology. The first centres on the nature of the science of epidemiology. Specifically, there are various grounds for thinking that epidemiology is not the dispassionate reporting of neutral scientific facts about diseases; rather, it is a science that is informed by conceptual and evaluative commitments. These worries were explained and ways of meeting them were suggested. The second discussion centres on epidemiological practice, and identifies various ethical issues in the collection of epidemiological data, some of which are shared with other kinds of research, others of which are distinctive. Finally, one illustrative application of a moral theory, namely, virtue ethics, to both kinds of challenges to epidemiology was presented.

6 Health Concepts and Promotion

The previous chapter discussed a fundamental feature of public health, i.e., epidemiology, its scientific basis. The main focus of this chapter is another deep-lying issue, namely, the nature of health. What is health? To answer this will require reflecting on others in the same family of 'health concepts', such as disease, illness, well-being, dysfunction, disability and condition. The first section of this chapter dispels the suspicion that this is not an important question in public health. In the next two sections, two conceptual claims about the nature of health are made. The first conceptual claim is that we are in a dilemma about the nature of health, between what are called the positive and negative conceptions of health, because 'health' is ambiguous. The second conceptual claim is that, on both these conceptions of health, health is an evaluative concept. The practical impact of these conceptual claims is then discussed: the impact on public health practice in general is explained; the importance of the ambiguous nature of health for health promotion in particular is discussed; finally, problems for other kinds of public health activity are described.

Is the nature of health important in public health ethics?

Before getting into details, let's consider three understandable reactions to the debate about the nature of health. The first reaction is that this topic only relates to certain branches of health care, not to the field of public health. In particular, the nature of mental health and illness is notoriously contentious, but perhaps this is a special case that can be confined to the philosophy of psychiatry. There is something in this. Conceptual worries about the nature of health and disease are rooted in the debate about mental illness sparked off by the anti-psychiatry movement, which questioned whether there is such a thing as mental illness, as opposed to merely societal disapproval of certain patterns of cognition and behaviour, 'mental illness' being a conve-nient label to excuse abusive 'treatments' (Szasz 1960; Fulford 1989: 4ff.). The contentiousness of health, illness, and health judgements is obvious in the context of mental health, and much of the best recent literature on health concepts starts from the controversy around mental illness and psychiatric disorders, notably Fulford's (1989) anal-ysis of illness as action-failure (cf. McKnight 1998; Eavy 2000), and Megone's (1998) Aristotelian functionalist argument (cf. Thornton 2000 and the other papers in that edition of *Philosophy, Psychiatry, and Psychology*).

But it is a mistake to think that, because the debate about the nature of health is very pertinent to mental health, it is not important in the field of public health. For one thing, public health is about all aspects of the health of populations, including protecting and promoting good mental health, so the debate about the nature of health is as relevant to public health as mental health is. Much more importantly, it is not just the nature of mental health and illness that is contentious, because the nature of physical health and disease is just as contestable (Fulford 1989: 3–24). The point is nicely summed up by Hare: 'We shall never be clear about these disputes [about what is called "mental illness"] until we are clear about the meaning of the term "illness", *whether applied to mental or physical conditions*, and about its opposite "health", and its near synonyms "disease" and "disorder"' (Hare 1986: 174 [emphasis added]).

Furthermore, like mental health, public health by its very nature invites worries about the meaning of health. In clinical medicine, con-ceptual questions about health and illness can be answered largely by patient behaviour. For example, to a large extent, illnesses can be taken to be conditions that patients want treated. Conversely, we can get a long way by assuming that a healthy patient is one who does not present for treatment. But public health cannot leave such questions to clients, because it deals with asymptomatic populations. So, when it comes to defining health, the onus is more on the public health pro-fessional than on the client. This is borne out by the fact that public health specialties beg the question as to the nature of health. As we shall see, health promotion is a particularly clear example but, as we shall also see, the nature of health is pertinent to the other branches of public health, too.

This might elicit a second reaction: is the nature of physical health, at least, not pretty obvious? Public health is about maintaining and improving health, and we all know what that means. Someone with bowel cancer is unhealthy; I myself, right now, am healthy. Again, there is something in this. There are clear-cut cases of being healthy and unhealthy. But we cannot conclude from these clear-cut cases that the meaning of health is uncontentious. The natures of justice, intelligence and freedom are not made uncontentious by the fact that there are clear-cut cases of injustice, unintelligence and lack of freedom. The problem with all such contested concepts is that, notwithstanding the clear-cut cases, we end up in a quandary when we try to develop a more general account of them. There is a typical dialectic. Someone suggests a definition of health (or another related health concept, such as disease or illness). This is then criticized using counter-examples that contradict the proffered definition. Then, the original definition is either reworked to accommodate the counter-example or substituted by another. Either way, the dialogue continues: another counter-example is presented, resulting in refinement or substitution, and so on (Hare 1986: 176ff.).

A third, more general reaction to this topic is that the analysis of health concepts is an academic (in the worst sense of the word) not practical matter. Again, there is something in this. Questions about the nature of health are no different in principle from questions about the nature of knowledge or causality, so they are bound to interest philosophers steeped in the business of conceptual analysis. But it is a mistake to conclude that the debate is merely academic. As Richard Hare puts it: 'The concept of health is one the understanding of which would help with both theoretical problems in philosophy *and practical problems in medicine*' (Hare 1986: 174 [emphasis added]). Generally speaking, we need to know what health is if we are going to devise and evaluate public health programmes to protect and enhance it. Relatedly, unless the nature of health is clarified, public health professionals could be working with different definitions of health, giving rise to an incoherent field comprising conflicting endeavours.

So, none of these three understandable reactions justifies scepticism about this topic. Nonetheless, each gives us something to bear in mind during the discussion. First, we need to keep public health in focus, as opposed to other branches of health care. Specifically, although we can borrow material from the debate about the nature of mental illness, we should be wary of getting embroiled in a discussion that is more relevant to psychiatric medicine than public health. Second, we must keep in mind that not all health judgements are contentious. Certain people are healthy whilst others are unhealthy on anyone's views on the nature of health. Nonetheless, disputes about the nature of health arise in, and influence, public health practice. Third, we must not get too academic, in the worst sense of the word. Our focus is on the practical implications of the contestable nature of health, not purely philosophical matters such as the fact–value distinction and the objectivity of values.

The key to discussing this topic further is to distinguish two related issues (Seifert and Taboada 2002: 241–5). The first is that 'health', as it is used in public health, can mean different things, or be defined in various ways. Specifically, 'health' can be conceived both negatively and positively. The second is about values and health: are values involved in the notion of health and health judgements, or are these value-free? It transpires that, on the understandings of health most prominent in public health, health is value-laden. For the sake of clarity, these two points are discussed separately in the next two sections; the last section of this chapter brings them back together to discuss how the debate about the nature of health impinges on public health practice.

First conceptual claim: 'health' is ambiguous

Turning to the first of the two issues just distinguished, there are two main views about the meaning of 'health'. The first is a negative view: to be healthy is to lack something. The most prominent suggestion is the biomedical conception of health, i.e., health is the absence of disease. So, someone is healthy when they are free of disease, and unhealthy if, and to the extent that, they have a disease. The second main view about the meaning of 'health' is positive: to be healthy is to have or be something. The most prominent contender is the well-being conception of health according to which someone is healthy when, and to the extent that, they enjoy well-being.

This distinction between negative and positive conceptions of health seems to figure largely in lay, as well as professional, conceptions of health and illness (Calnan 1987: 26ff.). And the biomedical and well-being conceptions are clearly connected because disease tends to compromise well-being. This might suggest that disease and well-being vary inversely with one another, with more disease equating to less well-being and less disease amounting to more well-being. Given this, absence of disease and well-being are not really two definitions of health; rather, they are two ways of describing a single health concept. But it is now well established in the literature that this is mistaken:

> ill health and well being cannot be related to each other as opposite poles on a linear scale. This approach has been tried by some theorists but it is not satisfactory, for it is logically possible (and not uncommon) for someone to have poor physical health but a high state of well being ... or a good state of physical health but poor well being. (Calman and Downie 2002: 394)

Absence of disease and well-being are discrete factors that can vary independently of one another. They are measured on discrete scales because the amount of well-being one has is independent of the extent to which one is disease-free, and vice versa. Let's look more closely at these two conceptions of health, in turn.

The negative conception of health

The negative conception of health as the absence of disease is a very intuitive account of the nature of health, one to which most people would naturally subscribe. Nonetheless, Campbell's (1990: 19) comment is still apposite: 'This traditional model is certainly not obsolete, as the problem of the prevention of the spread of AIDS ... graphically illustrates, but it is clearly inadequate.' The main reason for thinking it inadequate is that, whilst it is true that we often call someone with a disease 'unhealthy' and, conversely, someone free of disease 'healthy', we also use such terms in different, broader and more positive ways. The following is a typical illustration:

> A woman with multiple sclerosis who has come to terms with her condition and is leading a full and productive life within certain limitations might be viewed by some, including herself, as healthy. A man dying with bowel cancer who peacefully approaches his own death with the support of his family, might be said to have a very healthy approach despite the fact that his life is coming to an end. Conversely, someone who rarely feels happy, who is anxious, worried and lonely, although not suffering from an identifiable disease, may not be viewed as entirely healthy. It seems therefore that the biomedical conception would label some people as diseased whom we might wish to label healthy, and others healthy whom we might wish to label diseased in some sense. (Cribb and Dines 1993: 6)

It is worth pointing out a complication with these kinds of counter-examples to the biomedical model. Cribb and Dines have alluded to various things that can be healthy and unhealthy, including not only people, but also the lifestyle of the woman with multiple sclerosis, the bowel cancer victim's approach to death, and the mental condition of the person who rarely feels happy. So, the advocate of the biomedical conception of health can respond to their counter-examples as follows. Health is the absence of disease. The woman with multiple sclerosis herself, as a person, is unhealthy (she has a disease); on the other hand, she has a healthy attitude or lifestyle. This is not a counter-example because there is no one thing that is both healthy and diseased. The bowel cancer victim himself, as a person, is unhealthy (he has a disease); on the other hand, his approach to his predicament is healthy. Again, this is not a counter-example because no one thing is both healthy and diseased. Someone who rarely feels happy is a slightly more complicated case. Let's assume that they cannot be called mentally ill (their anxiety level is not that of an agoraphobic, for example). Then they, as a person, are healthy (they have no disease), though their lifestyle and cognitions may be unhealthy. Again, no counter-example: no one thing that is both healthy and diseased.

This caveat about their examples notwithstanding, the general point Cribb and Dines are making is a good one: the biomedical conception of health is simply too narrow to capture much of what we mean by 'health', as expressed in the way we actually use the word. Our use of the word suggests that we need an account of health in broader, more positive terms than mere disease absence. The disadvantage of the negative view of health is to the advantage of positive accounts.

The positive conception of health

Positive ways of construing health, such as the well-being conception, accommodate ordinary thought and talk about health that elude the biomedical account. Since, on the positive conception, health is no longer merely the absence of disease, someone with a disease can be healthy because they enjoy well-being, and someone without any disease can be unhealthy because they lack well-being.

What is wrong with positive accounts of health? The underlying problem is that we are in danger of defining one unclear concept, 'health', in terms of another equally opaque concept, 'well-being' (Seedhouse 1995; Buchanan 1995). There is a lack of both conceptual and practical clarity. Conceptually speaking, it is not clear whether well-being is to be thought of as an objective or subjective state. Can health experts judge the amount of well-being an individual has, because well-being is objectively discernible; or is well-being subjective and therefore dependent on individuals' self-assessment? The former smacks of health imperialism; the latter is a hostage to fortune because people value lots of states that health experts would not want to protect and promote. And, since life is capricious, on the well-being conception even the health status of a single individual would fluctuate with how their life happens to go; not only does this make a person's health status difficult to assess, it puts general pressure on the adequacy of the well-being view because we simply do not think that health status varies in this way. There are also practical problems. How are we to go about promoting well-being? Who has it, who does not? Is no one quite healthy because everyone could experience greater well-being? Or, might someone have just enough well-being to be healthy? But how much? Any quantification would seem arbitrary. And besides, the amount of well-being required to be healthy in one context will be different from the amount required in a different context.

Such difficulties with the positive conception of health as well-being can be illustrated by reference to the World Health Organization's (WHO) famous statement that health is a 'state of complete physical, mental and social well-being and not merely the absence of disease or infirmity' (World Health Organization 1948; cf. Buchanan 1995; van Spijk 2002; Buttiglione and Pasquini 2002). Quite what does, for example, 'physical well-being' amount to? This lack of clarity about well-being becomes even more obvious as one moves from the physical to other components in the WHO statement. What does mental well-being amount to; what is social well-being (Calman and Downie 2002: 394)? Does it depend on the objective judgement of health experts or the subjective assessments of individuals? Furthermore, WHO's list is not obviously complete. For example, spiritual and emotional experiences are constitutive of well-being for many people. Adding to the list adds murkiness; and a dilemma threatens between stipulating that the list is complete and indefinitely expanding it.

The dilemma between the negative and positive conceptions

The upshot of the discussion so far is that there is a dilemma about the nature of health between negative and positive accounts. So, it is not just a matter of thinking harder to decide which is the correct definition of health. This creates serious difficulties, as will be clarified in the next section. Beforehand, in this subsection, it is worth making a couple of comments, in passing, about the ambiguous nature of health.

First, there is a tendency in public health literature to exaggerate the point. Consider a fairly typical summary of the problematic nature of health: 'For some people health means not being ill, for others it means being fit or at the peak of physical condition, and for yet others it may mean being well adjusted, or content, or well balanced, or full of positive feelings of well-being, or even just happy' (Katz and Peberdy 1997: 89). Read at a glance, this seems like a very long list of definitions of health – eight, to be precise, padded out with phrases like 'yet others' – presented in a way that makes them sound quite incompatible. But this is somewhat exaggerated. Some of the definitions are close enough in meaning to be synonymous. For example, 'content' and 'happy' are clearly similar notions, as are 'well adjusted' and 'well balanced'. One or two of these putative definitions are simply unconvincing. 'Health' clearly does not mean 'happy' because these are quite different ideas (I can be healthy without being happy, and happy without being healthy). And the idea that health means 'at the peak of physical condition' is implausible. Professional athletes often say things like, 'I have a chance of gold if I can stay focused and healthy', but this is a metaphorical as opposed to literal use of 'healthy'.

When Katz and Peberdy's list is distilled down along these lines we end up with just the two (now familiar) sets of views. First, a negative conception of health, i.e., 'health means not being ill'; this is simply the biomedical conception of health as the absence of disease familiar from above. Second, a positive conception of health. Here there seem to be various plausible notions (well adjustedness, contentment). But note Katz and Peberdy's inclusion of 'well-being' here. Well-being is not another member of a list that includes such states as being content and well balanced. Rather, well-being is the umbrella term for all such positive health-related states (this is one of the reasons it is so unclear). So, it transpires that everything in Katz and Peberdy's list after 'health means not being ill' can be summed up as well-being. Hence, their list boils down to two views about the meaning of health – a negative definition of health as the absence of disease, and a positive view of health as well-being – which is not such a long, intimidating list after all. (Katz and Peberdy's is not an isolated case and there are other examples from the literature of this tendency to exaggerate how ambiguous health is: cf. Calman and Downie 2002: 393–4; Jones et al. 1997: 267ff.)

Another point of discussion is worth dwelling on for a moment. There are some worthy and sustained attempts in public health literature to develop definitions of health other than the standard negative and positive accounts. For example, according to the welfare conception of health suggested by Seedhouse (1986, 2004), health is the means to (or resources for, or foundations of) achieving goals. It is important to see that Seedhouse's definition is different from, and not a compromise between, the biomedical and well-being accounts of health. Both absence of disease and well-being are bases of definitions of health thought of as an end. By contrast, the welfare account suggests that health is not an end but a means. Specifically, the end is achieving one's life goals or potential, and health is the set of means necessary to attain this end. Typically, such means are said to include basic needs, including food and water; information, and personal abilities to assimilate it (such as literacy and numeracy); having, and being aware of one's duties towards, a community; and so on.

There are some very palatable aspects of Seedhouse's welfare conception. For one thing, there is a clear connection between welfare and health because, generally speaking, being ill compromises one's ability to achieve. Also, the welfare conception refocuses our attention on real-world determinants such as food and shelter, thereby suggesting a radical political agenda. For example, if health is the means to achieve, then the health agenda should include objectives such as freeing people from poverty. Nonetheless, the identification of health as the means to achieve seems intrinsically dubious. The general problem is that we do not readily think of being healthy as possessing the means to achieve our goals; rather, we think of health as an individual's state that is connected to, but independent of, welfare variables such as shelter and numeracy. We think that a rank underachiever can be healthy and, conversely, that someone who achieves all their life-goals can, nonetheless, be ill. So, being healthy, and having the means to achieve, are distinct things that can be pulled apart, both conceptually and practically speaking.

This is not intended as a detailed critique of Seedhouse's suggestion. Nonetheless, one rather telling point is worth flagging. For an advocate of the welfare conception to dig in their heels at this point and insist that being healthy is just having the means of achievement, is to run the risk of doing away with the very notion of health that is the point of their analysis. In other words, rather than combining the means of, or foundations for, achievement (things like food and shelter) and labelling the resultant amalgamation 'being healthy', it is much more natural to say that there are just those means (food, shelter, etc.); in which case, the welfare conception threatens to make redundant the very concept – i.e., 'health' – that it is supposed to elucidate.

Second conceptual claim: health is an evaluative concept

The previous section established the dilemma between two ways of construing health: negatively as the absence of disease, and positively as well-being (cf. Lavados 2002). Now we can move on to the second of the two conceptual claims distinguished at the outset of this chapter. Are health and health judgements value-neutral or value-laden; are they reports of empirical, scientific matters of fact, or value-judgements?

Let's work our way into this by expanding on this contrast between, on the one hand, the value-laden, evaluative or normative, and, on the other, the value-free, value-neutral or naturalistic. Although these rather loaded philosophical ideas are perhaps a little intimidating, we just need to get the gist rather than go deeply into them. Consider some of the things we might say about a painting. We might say, (1) the painting hangs in the Louvre, (2) the painting is very beautiful. Roughly, (1) is an example of a naturalistic claim, whereas (2) is an evaluative claim. The difference is that (2) contains a value term ('beautiful') whereas (1) is free of evaluative content (it does not contain an evaluative term). Relatedly, (1) is amenable to scientific investigation in the broad sense of observation and experience. In other words, (1) can be tested empirically, most obviously by going to the Louvre and checking what paintings hang there. By contrast, (2) is not amenable to verification by observation of that kind.

Health judgements are expressed in statements such as, 'he is in good health', 'she is in poor health', and 'the health of that population has improved'. Are such health judgements like (1) or (2)? Are they value-free, value-neutral descriptions of objective matters of fact about people and populations, or are they value-laden, evaluative claims? Of course, it depends on what you mean by health. So, let's recall from the previous section the two views most prominent in public health, the negative biomedical account of health as the absence of disease, and the positive account of health as well-being. Is health value-laden or value-free according to each of them?

Let's discuss the positive account of health as well-being first, because this is the less complicated of the two. It might seem obvious that health defined as well-being is evaluative because the notion of 'well-being' depends largely on values. It is easy to imagine one person who has one set of values being content when a different person in just the same condition is discontented because they have a different set of values. For example, a condition that restricts mobility would compromise the well-being of an active, athletic person more seriously than it would that of a more introverted, studious type of person. Conversely, the idea that well-being is quite independent of values systems seems very odd. Since well-being depends on what people value, on the view that health is well-being, health is evaluative. However, there is a complication to note here. The fact that it is easy to agree that health is value-laden on the well-being account does not preclude further disputes. Specifically, people might disagree about how the values involved are to be construed. For example, Englehardt (2002) and Donohue-White and Cuddeback (2002) agree that health is value-laden on the positive conception of health as well-being; but, because of their different views on the objectivity of the values involved, the former develops a 'post-modern' analysis whereas the latter presents an 'objectivist' account of health as well-being.

Leaving such complications aside, the point for our purposes is that it is easy to see that health is value-laden on the well-being account. What about the other main definition of health? The negative view of health as the absence of disease is more tricky because whether health is value-neutral on the biomedical account depends on whether 'disease' should be understood normatively or naturalistically. There is a very large literature on the nature of disease, and related concepts such as illness and dysfunction (Englehardt 1975; Reznek 1987; cf. Hesslow 1993; Khushf 1997). There is only space here for a brief sketch of this area rather than a thorough discussion. Broadly speaking, there are two main camps: the normativists who think disease is a value-laden concept, and naturalists who think it is value-free. The debate between these is quite well balanced in that there are good arguments on both sides. Räikkä (1996: 354) captures this well. On the one hand, he lists reasons for thinking that disease is a normative concept, namely, that health is desirable whilst disease is undesirable, what conditions count as diseases is culture-specific, and diseases are abnormalities. But, on the other hand, he immediately goes on to refer to the kinds of arguments in favour of naturalism about diseases, including both 'general objections, according to which *any* normative definition of "disease" is mistaken [and] specific objections against particular normativist arguments'.

Responses to this stand-off between normativists and naturalists about disease have made the topic very complicated. There are differences between views within the same camp. For example, some normativists about disease think objective values are at work (Lennox 1995) whilst other normativists think the relevant values are subjective

(Nordenfelt 1987; cf. Kovács 1998: 36; DeVito 2000: 547–51). There are those who think that absolutely everything about health and illness is value-laden: 'Not only "disease" but also such terms as "nerve" and "organ" are laden with conceptual values' (Stempsey 2000: 321). By contrast, in his analysis of mental disorders, Wakefield (1992a, 1992b) distinguishes a harm component, which is the evaluative aspect, and a value-free dysfunction component (cf. DeVito 2000: 551–60). Others combine normative and naturalistic elements, describing what DeVito (2000: 540) calls 'the inherently mixed (evaluative and value-neutral) nature of health and disease'. And the debate has refocused on concepts related to, but distinct from, that of disease, notably the concept of function. This is because the most common way of being a naturalist about disease is to be a functionalist: disease is functional failure, where function is understood in naturalistic, value-free terms (for example, the function of an organ is what it has evolved to do for the organism; cf. Nordenfelt 2003). The most famous exponent is Boorse, whose biostatistical theory eliminates values from the concept of disease (Boorse 1975, 1977, 1997; cf. DeVito 2000: 540–7; Stempsey 2000; Fulford 2001; Schaffner 1999). But some normativists retain the connection between disease and function by disagreeing that 'function' is value-free (Nissen 1993; McNally 2001; cf. Wakefield 2000).

Given this complexity and lack of space, let's assume that normativists about disease are correct in thinking that disease is a value-laden concept. This might seem a bit quick, but it reflects a discernible general trend in the literature away from value-neutral analyses of disease, such as Boorse's biostatistical theory, and towards increased recognition that values infuse our descriptions and ascriptions of disease states (cf. D'Amico 1998). More importantly, this assumption is a matter of being on the safe side. In other words, by assuming that normativism about disease is right, we make the negative conception of health as the absence of disease turn out to be a value-laden account of health. This is because, according to the biomedical model, health is the absence of disease, 'disease' – we are assuming – is an evaluative concept, so health is value-laden on the biomedical model. Better to make this assumption now, and deal with its impact on public health, than get lured into a false sense of security by thinking that naturalism about disease is right.

So, it transpires that health is an evaluative matter on both sets of views on the nature of health outlined in the previous section. It is worth pointing out that this is so even on other definitions of health that cannot be fully discussed here. Recalling Seedhouse's welfare conception of health as the means of achievement, for example, to say that health is the means to achieve life-goals or potential invites the question as to which life-goals and potentialities are relevant. It is obvious that life-goals reflect people's values: people with dissimilar values have different life-goals because what each is trying to do with their life depends on what they think matters (i.e., their values). The alternative, which is to say that certain life-goals are, as an objective matter of fact, the correct ones to go in for whatever people happen to think and feel about them, sounds very presumptuous. Since 'achievement' is a value-laden matter, health is value-laden according to the welfare conception.

The practical impact of the conceptual claims

To sum up the discussion so far, two conceptual claims have been made. First, there are two ways of defining health, negatively and positively. Second, on both, health is a value-laden concept. Why are these claims important to our present concerns, the practice of public health? Let's first state the practical implications and then discuss and illustrate them more fully.

Public health and the ambiguous nature of 'health'

The point of public health is to protect and enhance the health of populations. But there are different ways of understanding health. So, the field of public health might lack coherence. Different public health practitioners – individuals and institutions – might be aiming at different things because they interpret health differently. Relatedly, evaluating public health interventions becomes deeply problematic. One can only evaluate an activity against its aims and objectives. But different understandings of health usher in different aims and objectives. So, how successful an intervention is will be unclear. It would be a bit like saying the aim of a major corporation is to pursue success, without ensuring that there is a consensus on what 'success' means. The organization might well be incoherent, as individuals and departments set out to achieve what they understand success to be. And how successful they are is moot because it depends on what they are trying to achieve, which, in turn, depends on their definition of success.

There is a second practical implication of the conceptual claims made thus far. To introduce this, consider DeVito's (2000: 539) suggestion that 'if unrestricted values are allowed to infect our concepts of health and disease, then *anything* could be construed as healthy or diseased'. DeVito's idea is that health is evaluative, people can, and evidently do, value and disvalue myriad things, so any genuinely valued state turns out to be healthy and any genuinely disvalued state turns out to be unhealthy. Put like this, DeVito's claim is unconvincing. It is based on the assumption that as soon as values get involved, anything goes because values are merely subjective preferences: 'If judgements of mental illness are evaluations, expressions of values, rather than simply descriptions of facts, then mental illness cannot be an objective matter, a feature of the fabric of the world' (Thornton 2000: 75). But this assumption is very questionable. For one thing, there is a strong sense in contemporary philosophy that it is naïve to assume that the evaluative is subjective, whilst the non-evaluative is objective. Might not some values and value-judgements, at least, be objective? And this is borne out by more general reflection. Is it really feasible that longevity and being pain-free, for example, are mere subjective preferences?

But, though it is not convincing to think that, because of the evaluative nature of health, '*anything* could be construed as healthy or diseased', DeVito is on to something. Public health is about protecting and promoting health. Health, on the main ways it is understood in public health, turns out to be value-laden. Therefore, public health is about protecting and promoting certain values. The values may not be contentious (as mentioned, most people value longevity and disvalue pain, for example). But they can be, and often are. In other words, even if there are some objectively valuable things, such as longevity and being pain-free, there can be serious, legitimate and obstinate disagreements over other values. Specifically, the value system of a public health target population can differ markedly from that of health professionals, in two main respects. First, the value clients put on health – roughly, how important health is, relative to other goods – might be far lower than that assumed by public health professionals. Second, the values people have, which differ from those of the health establishment, might mean that 'lay conceptions' of health are in play that differ markedly from the understanding of health shared by health professionals (Calnan 1987: 17–40).

In such circumstances, how would public health activities in general – and health promotion advice and initiatives in particular – appear to a target population? They will seem to be the expression and imposition of alien views about what is valuable, what matters, what is significant and worthwhile. Consequently, public health initiatives that make perfect sense given health establishment values will not be well received by clients who have a different set of values. Understandably, members of the target population would retort in such terms as, 'what makes you think you know what's best for me?' and 'why are you imposing your value system on me?' The fact that interventions intended to promote alien values and alien conceptions of health are typically backed up by serious State power will only deepen the resentment. Public health comes to seem like health fascism. The upshot is likely to be recalcitrance on the part of the target population, and frustration on the part of professionals convinced that they are in the right.

Let's pursue this theme by illustrating the practical impact of the analysis of health concepts, by focusing on a major branch of public health, namely, health promotion. First, some preparatory remarks.

What is 'health promotion'?

Cribb comments that 'it is notoriously difficult to pin down the idea of health promotion' (1995: 199). He goes on to allude to 'the ambiguity of the term "health promotion", and the confusion about its borders' (p. 205). Cribb's comments are typical in that most texts on the ethics of health promotion start by acknowledging that its nature and definition are problematic. Hence, there are numerous attempts to analyse the concept of health promotion (Nordenfelt 1995), and various lists of taxonomies, approaches and models for health promotion (Naidoo and Wills 2000). This feature of health promotion is not shared by other public health measures, such as immunization and screening, and has generated some interesting and contentious literature (Seedhouse 2004). The key to understanding why health promotion is considered hard to define is to distinguish the two problems to which Cribb alludes. The first is the important one for our purposes, so let's deal quickly with the second.

The second problem in defining health promotion to which Cribb alludes is the 'confusion about its borders', i.e., the problem of how to set a boundary between the profession of health promotion and all other health-promoting activities. Myriad activities are health promoting. Any attempt at a taxonomy of health-promoting activities would be futile because of their sheer range and variety. All of health care is health promoting, from the initiatives implemented by specialist health promoters in the name of health promotion, through preventive measures, such as immunization and screening, to curative medicine and high-tech surgery. Health is promoted by legislation, regulation, and activities initiated outside of the health sector without the express intention of promoting health, such as transport policy and community development. Health is also promoted as a by-product of other, apparently quite unconnected, activities. Plumbers promote health when they fix a toilet. Parents promote health when they put coats on their children on a windy day. Football coaches promote health when they make their team do exercises. One's next meal, and even one's next breath, are health promoting.

On the one hand, we could define health promotion to include everything that is health promoting. The advantage of this is that it does not leave out anything important. But it is too broad a definition to be useful (cf. Cribb and Dines 1993: 26–7). On the other hand, we might distinguish health-promoting activities that belong in the sub-category, health promotion. For example, we might restrict health promotion to health-promoting activities undertaken by professional health promotion experts, or which intentionally aim at promoting health, or which promote health directly as opposed to indirectly. Such a distinction would afford a clear, specific, manageable and useful definition of the profession of health promotion. But any such restriction seems arbitrary and begs the question as to why such-and-such a feature – and, hence, such-and-such types of health-promoting activities – are the important ones. Furthermore, it risks ignoring important health-promoting activities that happen to fall outside the stipulated boundary.

This dilemma reappears in various guises throughout the literature. To illustrate, consider a comment by Nordenfelt (1995: 185):

> By health promotion I mean something very general. I incorporate all measures performed by a particular individual A with the intention of maintaining or improving the health of some individual B, where A and B can, but need not, be identical persons. An important exception from this general characteristic [of health promotion] is, however, made: I am not concerned with curative medical health care.

The dilemma as it emerges in Nordenfelt's comment is: either we allow Nordenfelt's 'exception', i.e., his restricting health promotion to the non-curative, which would result in a manageable set of activities, but which, given his definition of health promotion, is simply question-begging; or we disallow his 'exception', in which case we avoid begging the question as to why curative medical care is ruled out, but then 'health promotion' means the whole of health care, which is too wide a definition to be useful.

How important is this boundary problem? It would be a bad idea simply to deny the point: we do need to restrict ourselves to a manageable topic, but cannot do so without placing a seemingly arbitrary boundary around some health-promoting activities. But defining any set of activities is tricky. Health promotion is no worse off in this regard than any other interesting profession. For example, economics, education and politics all suffer from the same complaint: from amongst all those activities that are economic, educative and political, where is the boundary around the fields of economics, education, politics? The same dilemma between allowing too much in, and imposing an arbitrary restriction, arises. These other professions do not seem to be breast-beating about being only vaguely delineated. Perhaps health promotion should accept that there is no one defining characteristic of all the activities that belong to the profession, and that health promotion shades off into other similar sets of activities, such as public policy making, community development and criminal justice. There cannot be a watertight definition; nonetheless, we need not be intimidated by this because we have a firm enough grasp on what comprises the profession (cf. Seedhouse 1995: 66–7).

Furthermore, at this point, advocates of health promotion might turn things on their head by insisting that, far from being problematic, the fact that 'health promotion' is vague in the way just discussed is a positive thing. Specifically, the fact that health promotion is such a broad, open-ended profession facilitates a more radical health agenda. Lots of concerns can be included under the banner of health promotion – from smoking cessation to community development to poverty eradication – precisely because we are not dogmatic about what is being promoted, and about there being a fixed, rigid boundary between health promotion and the health promoting. What is so bad about a profession that self-consciously recognizes its vagueness and fluidity, and thereby develops a multi-faceted, and consequently more radical, agenda (Cribb and Dines 1993: 20–33; Cribb and Duncan 2002: 6–17; cf. Yeo 1993: 226–7; Seedhouse 2004)?

Health promotion and the ambiguous nature of health

The more important problem for present purposes is the first to which Cribb alludes: 'the ambiguity of the term "health promotion".' In other words, 'health promotion' is ambiguous because, as clarified above, 'health' is ambiguous. As McCormick (1996: 620) dryly comments in a classic piece: 'Those who are keen to promote the public health seldom define the nature of the health that is their concern.' Even if they do, '[g]iven that there are multiple, and often competing, accounts of what is meant by "health", there will be analogous disputes about the purposes (and in turn, therefore, the processes) of health promotion' (Cribb and Duncan 2002: 145). This seems to be a serious problem for a number of reasons.

At worst, since 'health' is ambiguous, perhaps health promotion is a fragmentary, incoherent profession lacking focus and direction, with health promoters that understand 'health' in one way in conflict with health promoters that understand 'health' differently. On a negative account of health, health promotion means promoting the absence of disease. The onus will be on health promoters helping people to avoid contracting disease, i.e., on reducing the incidence and prevalence of disease. Health promotion will comprise familiar kinds of specialist health promotion activities implemented by health promotion experts, such as anti-smoking campaigns and healthy-eating programmes. But, on a positive conception of health, health promotion means enhancing well-being. This suggests a wider agenda than that typified by getting people to avoid lung cancer by smoking less, because it implies a conception of how people should, in much more general terms, live their lives. When someone says, 'I'm a health promoter', what do they mean? It depends on what they are promoting. But this could, quite legitimately, be any one of a number of things, depending on which meaning of 'health' is in play.

To reiterate, the problem is not simply that of being clearer. The problem is that, since the meaning of 'health' is ambiguous, what health promotion is, is contestable. This ushers in the related problem that, since the nature of health is contentious, and there is no consensus on the aims of health promotion, interventions cannot be properly evaluated. A health intervention can only be evaluated against its goals. For example, the goal of an anti-smoking health promotion campaign is to make people healthy in the sense of disease-free, the success of the campaign being evaluated by looking at how many clients quit. But someone who thinks of health in a more positive way might disagree. They might say that, though the campaign is successful on its own terms, it is not a success in general because health is not the absence of disease. In order to justify health promotion, we have to be clear that what health promotion promotes is worthwhile, which again requires knowing what is being promoted in the first place (Buchanan 1995).

How deep is the problem?

How big a problem is the ambiguous nature of 'health' to health promotion? Is it disastrous for the profession because it results in serious confusion and incoherence? One reason for thinking not is that the ambiguity in 'health' seems to boil down to just two sets of views, i.e., negative versus positive accounts of health (recall the way that the problem as to the nature of health tends to be exaggerated in health promotion literature, and the criticism of Seedhouse's alternative conception). Each account captures something important in what we mean by calling someone healthy. It is not at all obvious that the accounts are always or inevitably incompatible. So, rather than jettisoning one definition of health in favour of the other, perhaps we should retain both conceptions. The obvious objection is that we do not end up with a single, univocal definition of health, nor, therefore, 'health promotion'. But this is a theoretical problem that can be avoided by simply giving up this hope of finding univocal definitions of health concepts. In sum, health promoters can promote both the absence of disease and well-being.

According to the literature, any such attempt to make negative and positive accounts of health compatible is hopeless because 'various formulations [of the concept of health], although they may be internally coherent, are not mutually compatible' (Buchanan 1995: 223). But this is worth dwelling on a bit. It depends on what one means by compatibility. As just stated, there is one important sense in which the biomedical and well-being conceptions of health really are incompatible: conceptually speaking, they are incompatible definitions of health. In other words, since freedom from disease and well-being are independent health variables that cannot be placed on the same continuum, conceptually speaking, negative and positive conceptions of health are incompatible. But are they incompatible, practically speaking? Sometimes, it is simply assumed in the literature that they are. To illustrate, consider an example from Jones et al. (1997: 268) involving a group of unemployed 16–18-year-old school leavers who 'spend much of their time watching television, hanging out together, smoking, drinking, and playing slot machines'. Jones et al. present a challenge to a health promotion team: what are the team's priorities in terms of promoting the group's health, and what grounds their list of priorities? Jones et al. want to suggest that there are deep problems for health promoters here because of the ambiguous nature of health: 'it is a very difficult question indeed. The danger is not so much one of superficial disagreement but one of superficial agreement obscuring really substantial differences' (p. 268).

But is this right? Why not think of the health of members of this small population as both the absence of disease and well-being, and work to protect and promote their health in both senses? Health promoters might well worry about the smoking because health is the absence of disease and smoking is a risk factor for various diseases. And health promoters might well worry about the group's use of their leisure time, partly because health is the absence of disease and this sedentary lifestyle is a risk factor for various diseases; and largely because there are healthier – in a different sense (the positive, well-being sense) – ways young people can spend their time. So, health promoters might offer health education around smoking and alcohol and, at the same time, lobby for a community resource such as a football pitch or basketball park. There are good grounds for both. Doing the one does not preclude the other. Perhaps the difficulty is not so great after all: we aim to minimize disease and maximize well-being.

Critics of this line of thought will insist that, though it may be possible in principle to promote both the absence of disease and well-being, we can predict the inevitable practical problems. The obvious example is that there are resources to implement either the smoking cessation service or the community development project, but not both. How, then, is the team to prioritize? Which is more important: to use the scarce resources to combat the smoking, or to attempt something more to do with well-being in the broader and more positive sense? Of course, this can be a really intractable problem. But are there 'really substantial differences' being obscured here? After all, as Jones et al. say (p. 267), concerning health, welfare, and well-being, '[o]f course these positions are not entirely discrete and will tend to merge into one another in theory and in practice'. And this seems right; there is not the ideological stand-off these authors would have us envisage; rather there is a team of health promoters who understand the complexity of the situation and aim to develop interventions that will maximize the use of their scarce resources.

This is not to deny that tensions can arise within a health promotion team between (a) adherents to the biomedical account of health and (b) adherents to the well-being account of health. For example, group (a) might prefer to spend a budget on a machine to check cholesterol with a view to reducing incidence of heart disease, whereas group (b) wants to spend the same budget on a community-strengthening project. But, to reiterate, how deep is the disagreement here? Do (a) and (b) have different health goals? Or do they share the same complex goal – absence of disease and more well-being – whilst trying to achieve them using somewhat different, and complementary, styles and methods? Probably, both sets of health promoters think that a poor diet and heart disease are sources of illness. Group (a) focuses on the threat of disease; group (b) focuses on the threat to well-being. But both groups have the same general aims. Group (a) tends to use 'harder' methods such as target-setting, quantifiable gains, and fairly standard techniques such as health education; group (b) tends to use 'softer' methods such as community involvement in project design, and a more holistic approach. But this is not a deep dispute about the nature of health promotion based on different understandings of health; rather, it is a matter of two groups trying to achieve the same goals, albeit in a different style, using different methods (cf. Downie 1990: 3–6; Jones et al. 1997: 266–8).

Perhaps this is all too sanguine. Consider a different case, one presented by Ewles and Simnett (1995: 35) and discussed in Katz and Peberdy (1997: 99–100), centring on an 'overweight, middle-aged, unemployed patient'. What kind of health promotion would be appropriate for such a patient? Specifically, what should the health advice to that patient be, concerning their raised blood pressure and alcohol intake? Again, these authors want to suggest that the answers, depending as they do in large part on the issues under discussion in this chapter, are very obscure: it depends on what one means by health. On a negative conception of health as the absence of disease, the important thing is the raised blood pressure, which is a risk factor for all kinds of diseases. Reducing alcohol intake can be expected to lower the patient's blood pressure and therefore reduce the risk of disease. So, the doctor ought to persuade the patient to drink less. But, on a conception of health as well-being, things look different. Given the patient's circumstances, it might well be that going to the pub or bar to drink beer is vital to maintaining their levels of well-being. Stopping drinking – even compromising the pleasure of drinking by harping on about its detrimental effects – might well be disastrous for the patient's well-being. So, on this account of health it would be dubious of the doctor to persuade the patient to drink less.

Again, though, one might want to say more. The way the case is presented, the doctor is left with a straight choice between recommending drinking and not drinking. But life is rarely this straightforward. Better, surely, to think of two compatible goals here, i.e., avoiding diseases and enjoying well-being. Given this, various health-promoting measures offer a compromise between the two. The doctor might recommend some, but less, drinking. Or they might recommend alternative strategies: lots of drinking but more exercise and regular health checks, too.

This discussion as to how deeply the ambiguous nature of health affects the practice of health promotion could be continued, but there is not space here. Let's leave it at this point. It would not be surprising if the doctor in the previous scenario, steeped in the medical model and feeling responsible for the patient's physical condition, thinks that the important thing is their patient's raised blood pressure. What matters from their perspective is the increased risk of disease and the ameliorating effects of drinking less. But the important thing – what matters – from the patient's perspective might well be social, not physical: the camaraderie amongst the drinkers at the pub or bar, and the sense of inclusion and involvement. The doctor thinks it is unhealthy to drink so much. The patient thinks, 'Sit around the flat all day moping about being unemployed? Now that would be really unhealthy.' Neither is wrong; it is just that they are subscribing to different accounts of health based on different sets of values.

Other public health activities

The ambiguous nature of health causes problems that are especially acute, and well documented, in health promotion. But it would be a mistake to think that the contestable nature of health is important only in this branch of public health. The fact that the nature of health is contentious matters to the whole of public health. For example, epidemiology, the study of diseases, is the scientific basis of public health. How can we do epidemiology without knowing what to study? And how can we know what to study without first knowing what a disease is, which, in turn, requires our saying what health is? Should we be doing the epidemiology of so-called 'social diseases'? Should we be doing the epidemiology of health behaviours? How do we prioritize between different conditions when epidemiological research resources are scarce? It depends on what we are trying to achieve, i.e., on what health is.

The same goes for screening. In public health, we screen for diseases to protect and promote health. But what should we screen for? The answer can seem obvious: we should screen people for diseases in order to promote health. But disease and health are value-laden terms that are open to different interpretations. So, there will be screening programmes that are contentious because they are based on contestable assumptions about the nature of disease and health. For example, we screen foetuses for Down's syndrome. But is Down's syndrome a disease? Can a Down's syndrome child be healthy or not? Is the notion of a healthy Down's syndrome child oxymoronic? If so, every Down's syndrome child is ill or unhealthy, which raises the question as to what to say when such a child becomes ill due to other conditions. What about screening for social disease? Should health professionals screen their patients for domestic abuse? Has this got anything to do with health? Perhaps it can be justified on the negative view of health because domestic abuse is a risk factor for various injuries. But it would not be surprising if a GP were to decline to implement such a screening programme on the grounds that he or she is a health professional, and domestic abuse is not a health matter. It depends on what you mean by 'health'.

Immunization is interesting in this regard. The point of immunization programmes is to control or eradicate disease. This seems straightforward because immunization programmes tend to be focused on clear-cut cases of disease. Of course, this point applies to epidemiology and screening too: we are justified in researching the aetiology of, and screening for, clear-cut cases of conditions that are diseases. But epidemiology and screening become contentious on different accounts of health, when we move away from the clear-cut. By contrast, there does not seem to be the same sense that mass immunization programmes become controversial because their justification depends on what meaning of health is in play. Nonetheless, it would be wrong to conclude that the contestability of health is irrelevant to mass immunization. Suppose there is a contest over scarce resources and we can fund either a vaccination programme or a health promotion programme. Suppose the health promotion programme is based on a broad and positive conception of health; for example, it consists of a community-strengthening scheme. One kind of objection to funding the latter rather than the former is that the former is the real health issue. It would be good to do both, but since health is really the absence of disease, and the immunization programme is designed to combat a disease, that should be our priority. But a health promoter working with a broader, more positive conception of health would demur. Again, it depends on what we are trying to achieve, which, in turn, depends on what we mean by health.

Concluding remarks

Two main conceptual claims have been made in this chapter: there is more than one adequate understanding of health; and, on the definitions of health pertinent to public health, health is a value-laden notion. This gives rise to practical problems. When it comes to evaluating public health interventions, we have to ask two questions. Quite what is being protected and promoted by such-and-such an intervention; i.e., what meaning of 'health' is in play? And what – and whose – values are being reflected in such-and-such an intervention; ones that can be defended and justified, or ones that are glibly assumed to be important and universal? Although such questions apply most obviously to health promotion, it has been demonstrated that they impact on other kinds of public health activity.

7 Health Promotion as Behaviour Modification

The topic of the previous chapter is the ambiguous and value-laden nature of health. A major theme that developed there is the impact of this on health promotion. This chapter pursues this theme by discussing the other main concern about health promotion in public health ethics, namely, the ethics of behaviour modification. The first section of this chapter provides more details about health promotion as behaviour modification. This involves responding to two worries about this focus on behaviour modification: first, that it smacks of victim-blaming; second, that it is epistemically insecure. The rest of the chapter discusses the ethics of behaviour modification techniques. In the middle section, the main ways by which health promoters try to modify behaviours, and the ethical issues they raise, are sketched. In the third and final section, the most important grounds for justifying interventions intended to change health behaviours are discussed.

Health promotion as behaviour change

To introduce the idea of health promotion as behaviour modification, consider a comment by Leichter:

> There is now widespread agreement among both the general population and health professionals that a good deal of disease is self-inflicted, the

product of our own imprudent behaviour. The premise that individuals contribute significantly to their own ill health or premature death appears unassailable in view of the mounting evidence relating various personal habits and lifestyle choices, such as poor nutrition, smoking, alcohol and drug abuse, failure to wear seat belts, and unsafe sexual practices, to major causes of morbidity and mortality. (Leichter 1991: xiii)

As Leichter points out, it is now common knowledge that health status is in part the effect of behaviours. So, a way to maintain and improve health is to modify those health behaviours. This is the distinctive feature at the heart of the ethics of health promotion: health promoters aim to modify health behaviours in order to maintain and improve health status.

This is not to smuggle in a definition of health promotion: 'health promotion' cannot being defined as behaviour modification, because we cannot reduce the profession to attempts to modify health behaviours. For example, Naidoo and Wills (2000) consider behaviour change to be one of five types of health promotion. And let's also recall the point from the previous chapter that it is not a good idea to go in for watertight definitions of health promotion but, rather, to take health promotion to be an inclusive and rather fluid subspecialty. So, whilst this is not to define health promotion, the point is that, in discussing the ethics of health promotion, the most interesting and contentious issues arise when health promoters attempt to modify behaviours.

Further details

To flesh out this notion of health behaviours, various related factors need to be distinguished. Consider smoking. A smoker likes, prefers or desires to smoke. A smoker chooses, or decides, to smoke. A smoker acts, or behaves, in a certain way. A smoker's smoking might be part of their lifestyle that includes other risk-taking and macho behaviours. For the sake of convenience, 'health behaviours' and 'behaviour modification' are used in this chapter as umbrella terms to include all these elements. There are not sharp boundaries between these aspects of health behaviours because preferences, choices, actions and lifestyles shade into one another (Veal 1993; Nordenfelt 1995: 187–9). Relatedly, someone might stop smoking because they stop wanting to smoke in the first place; because, though they want to smoke, they choose not to do so; because, though they want and choose to smoke, they cannot act on their decision (cigarettes are priced out of their reach, for example); or because they undergo a lifestyle shift that makes smoking seem inappropriate.

Health promoters intervene to alter all these aspects of health behaviours. This is worth noting because the ethics of changing behaviours depends in part on which aspect is being targeted. There seems to be a continuum from less to more controversial interventions. 'Nudging' people towards healthy options is presented as an uncontroversial strategy because it leaves people free to choose unhealthily, as discussed in Chapter 4. Generally, interventions that target a discrete behaviour, such as wearing a seatbelt and putting one's baby 'back to sleep', are considered to be less controversial because they home in on one action and leave everything else as it is. Targeting people's desires and preferences seems more controversial because it attempts to change them (i.e., people) as opposed to their actions. Attempts to modify whole lifestyles are most controversial because they raise some very deep questions about how one should live one's life; as philosophers put it, what is the good life for a human being? One might well wonder whether governments are best placed to answer this.

A practical point about these different facets of health behaviours is that the direction of influence can vary between them. For example, changing preferences often results in a behaviour change; conversely, though less obviously, changing behaviours can result in a preference change. Let's take each of these in turn. Many of the behaviour modification techniques discussed in this chapter attempt to change preferences in order to change behaviours. For example, social marketing attempts to manipulate preferences by changing the image or perception of smoking. Other techniques attempt to change behaviours in order to change preferences. For example, an assumption behind restrictive practices is that taking away the means to indulge in an unhealthy behaviour will have the result that people will stop wanting to indulge in the first place.

Is the distinction between behaviour and other factors that influence health as clear as being implied here? Is not behaviour always relevant to morbidity and mortality? Take one possible point of contrast: we might assume that some illness is due to behaviours, some due to accidents. But behaviour is always relevant to an accident; for example, the road traffic accident victim had to be behaving in a certain way in order to get knocked down. Perhaps this still leaves factors that are obviously non-behavioural, such as illness due to one's genetic complement. But, presumably, even here there is at least some behavioural element in that a person in one environment living one way will have a different disease pattern from another with the same genetic characteristic who lives in a different way in a different environment.

In response to this worry it is useful to dwell on two of Leichter's phrases. First, 'imprudent behaviour' implies that, at least in some sense, the fact that certain behaviours relate to illness is common knowledge (i.e., at least to the extent that it is appropriate to call the behaviour in question 'imprudent'). The victims themselves might not have this knowledge; nonetheless, it is common knowledge, so it can be said of them that they are acting imprudently. For example, the connection between smoking and lung cancer, and between unsafe sex and HIV, is now common knowledge in this sense. Second, Leichter's phrase, 'personal habits and lifestyle choices', suggests that the behaviours in question are habitual, well-established behaviour patterns, not one-off events. For example, 'smoker' in this context refers to someone who smokes regularly, not someone who only has a cigar on their birthday. So, the idea is that health status is influenced by patterns of behaviour that are imprudent because they are known to relate to morbidity and mortality. Now we have the contrast with other factors. For example, the road traffic accident victim might have been indulging in a 'personal habit and lifestyle choice' (for example, they always walk that way to work because they like the view) but were not acting 'imprudently' (it is not common knowledge that walking that way to work causes morbidity and mortality).

Referring again to his quote, Leichter emphasizes the negative relationship between behaviours and health status, i.e., that imprudent health behaviour is associated with disease (for example, smoking is associated with lung cancer). In fact, the connection between behaviours and health status is both negative and positive. The positive aspect of the relationship is that certain behaviours conduce to health improvements amongst those who are basically well. For example, moderate exercise improves the health of people who are not, and are not likely to become, unwell. So, the relevant feature in health promotion is the attempt to maintain and improve health status by manipulating health behaviours, where these can be negative (health compromising) or positive (health enhancing).

Given this, behaviour modification is a feature of health promotion whether one prefers the narrow and negative biomedical account of health or the broad and positive well-being conception of health, which were discussed in the previous chapter. Regarding a negative construal of health, sometimes the aim of health promotion is to dissuade people from behaviours that put them at risk of disease. For example, health promoters motivate people to give up smoking in order to avoid lung cancer. Regarding a positive construal of health, sometimes the aim of a health promotion campaign is to encourage behavioural changes intended not only to avoid risks of disease but also to promote well-being. For example, health promoters motivate people to exercise regularly, partly as a preventive measure, but also because they will thereby feel less stressed and more contented.

Victim-blaming

One problem with making behaviour modification the focus of a discussion of the ethics of health promotion is that it smacks of victim-blaming. To explain, we need a potted history of health promotional thinking. This is bound to be very quick and miss out on many details (MacDonald 2002). Also, this theme could have been introduced in other ways, such as by reference to the critique of the 'health belief model' (Roden 2004). Nonetheless, a good place to start is the Lalonde Report (Lalonde 1974), an influential response to the then growing sense of inadequacy of the medical model of health. The report helped clarify the importance of non-clinical factors in health status. Specifically, Lalonde argued that health is in part a factor of individuals' behaviour patterns. This ushered in an era in which health promotion was understood as promoting healthy lifestyles.

Lalonde was subjected to a structural critique consisting of pointing out the numerous problems with the assumption that individuals are to blame for their own illness (Veatch 1980; Marantz 1990; Yeo 1993). It is conceptually flawed because an individual is not a free-floating entity whose lifestyle can be understood and explained in isolation from the factors beyond their control – upbringing, culture, society, wealth status, genome, etc. – that mould them. It is wrong to think that people are free to choose healthier options, because such factors, which are outside of the individual's control, determine their behaviours. (This echoes the communitarian critique of liberal individualism, as discussed in Chapter 4.) Hence, 'the assignment of responsibility to individuals who suffer from deteriorated health and premature death due to behaviours not of their own choosing is a form of blaming the victim, a second punishment with social disapproval for those who have already been punished by circumstances' (Dougherty 1995: 213). Additionally, to focus on individual behaviours is to draw attention away from the main determinants of health, which are not dubious personal decisions but large-scale environmental factors (this recalls the mass sanitation programmes in the nineteenth-century public health heyday). And the stress on individual behaviours is politically dubious in appearing to vindicate State reluctance to address the real causes of ill-health, including macro-level socio-economic structures.

The upshot was the 'new health promotion' (or 'new public health'), a central plank in which was the Ottawa Charter for Health Promotion (1986), which gave expression to the structural critique by describing a social model for health and an agenda for social and health reform. This was wide-ranging and radical. It viewed health, health status and the determinants of health through a wide-angled lens, bringing into view environmental factors, including not only the physical, but also the social, cultural, economic, etc., contexts of people's lives. And, relatedly, it was radical in insisting that any serious attempt at health promotion has to work on these environmental factors and not focus just on individuals and their lifestyles. Generally, the importance in health promotion of reflection on, and reform of, wider societal structures was established.

It will be useful to label the two factors in play here: (a) individuals' freely chosen health behaviours, and (b) background factors (such as genetic complement and socio-economic positioning) that are not chosen. Lalonde seemed to focus on (a); the structural critique insists that the real cause of ill health is (b); so, to focus overmuch on (a) is victim-blaming; reflecting this, the new public health focuses on (b). Our problem is that, in this chapter, behaviour modification is taken to be central to health promotion ethics; i.e., the focus is on (a). This might seem to miss the point of the structural critique, so it might seem naïve in the way Lalonde came to be seen as naïve, i.e., in blaming individuals for their illness when really they are victims of macro-level influences that are not a matter of choice. How might this worry be met?

Avoiding the charge of victim-blaming

One approach is to try to reinstate the importance of freely chosen behaviours to one's health. Two philosophical ways of attempting this are as follows. First, a conceptual analysis of responsibility (and related notions such as liability and culpability) might reveal that individuals can be held responsible for their health more than the new public health suggests. The second is to enter the debate about free-will and moral responsibility: it might be that we can establish that individuals are substantially free to behave as they do, can be held responsible for their health behaviours and so are (at least largely) to blame for their illness. But these kinds of approaches are unpromising. Dworkin (1981) is a good example of the former; but what is striking about his analysis of responsibility is that, for all its subtlety, when it comes to the practical business of policy application, it raises more questions than it answers. As for getting into the metaphysics of free-will: 'Understood as a problem of metaphysics, as the freedom versus determinism debate, there is little hope for resolution ... The history of Western philosophy is testament to the perennial character of this dispute' (Dougherty 1995: 216).

So, we need a better way of meeting the worry that focusing on behaviour modification smacks of victim-blaming. Dougherty (1995) distinguishes the 'freedom model' from a 'facticity model'. His point is that both models contain insights. The insight in the freedom model is that, to some extent, people are free to choose healthier behaviours, so are partly responsible for their health status; in turn, it is worthwhile praising, blaming, taking responsibility for, and trying to modify their preferences. The insights in the facticity model are that macro-level factors mitigate some behaviours, and to focus solely on individual behaviours is to miss out on massive opportunities for health gain afforded by macro-level developments. Dougherty's point is that, since both contain important insights, neither model can be jettisoned. Eschew the freedom model and we fail to motivate individuals to choose more healthily; eschew the facticity model and we miss out on health gain by macro-level developments. Furthermore, practically speaking, they are compatible. So, we can hold both that people are responsible for some of their behaviours and resultant health status, and that macro-level factors influence people and their health. He recommends reconciling the two models by clarifying and retaining both.

Putting this reconciliatory project into historical terms, the development of health promotion, as illustrated by the shift from the Lalonde Report to the Ottawa Charter, does not excise behaviour modification from the health promotion agenda. Rather, it amounts to recognizing that macro-level societal and environmental factors influence an individual's behaviours. In other words, the structural critique does not deny that behaviours affect health but, rather, develops that insight by insisting on taking into account the factors and forces that mould, explain, and therefore mitigate relevant behaviours. So, generally speaking, there is not the tension between old-style health promotion as promoting healthy lifestyles, and the new, sophisticated public health that contextualizes individuals, sometimes suggested in the literature (MacDonald 2002: 36–7). And, more specifically, since both perspectives contain vital insights, the focus in this chapter on individual health behaviours is warranted.

The epistemology of health behaviour modification

The point of the previous subsection is that we can focus on health promotion as behaviour modification and avoid the charge of victim-blaming. But there is another very general problem with this topic worth dealing with here. Health promotion as behaviour modification raises various epistemological concerns.

The key here is to distinguish two epistemic problems about behaviour modification. The first, more obvious one is that claims about the effects of behaviours on health are never as secure as one would like. Relatedly, it is familiar for the public to be impatient with health advice because it is liable to change ('One minute they tell you it's good for you, the next it's bad' and so on). This is part of the general point that epidemiological evidence underdetermines causal claims in health. This was discussed in Chapter 5, where it was argued that scepticism about epidemiology is less convincing than is often suggested:

> Though epidemiologists and public health officials debate the finer points of such studies, there is little question that they are significant. Individually and collectively we might do much to alter the morbidity statistics of the populations in the advanced industrial world if we were able to change behavior. (Bayer 1981: 26)

There is a second, less obvious epistemological problem. Whether we should run a health promotion programme depends in part on its effectiveness in terms of influencing behaviours and thereby improving health status. It is easy to assume that we can verify the effectiveness of a health promotion programme. But we can only do one of two things: implement it or not. So we only know how people behave having run the programme, or how people behave having not run the programme. What we can never do is compare behaviour patterns with, and behaviour patterns without, the health promotion intervention. This seems to imply that we cannot verify the intervention's effectiveness. Therefore, it appears, health promotion is never justified: 'all health promotion interventions which have not been sufficiently evaluated ought to be treated as medical research addressed to the population' (Tountas et al. 1994: 850; cf. Cribb and Duncan 2002: 81–98; International Union for Health Promotion and Education 1999).

How strong is this argument? Consider two ways we might defend health promotion. First, we might note that the same problem applies to just about everything in health care. We can never be certain of the effectiveness of my trip to the dentist because we can never compare the state of my teeth having made the trip with the state of my teeth having not made the trip. Nonetheless, we think it a good idea to go to the dentist. Second, we might invoke the utilitarian distinction between actual and expected utility, as explained in Chapter 1. The epistemological problem is that we cannot be certain about the actual utility of a behaviour modification programme. But we can still calculate its expected utility and, according to the way utilitarianism was presented in Chapter 1, morality is a matter of maximizing expected utility. So, provided we are confident that a programme of behaviour modification will maximize expected utility, we have a utilitarian justification for going ahead.

But a sceptic about health promotion would respond by suggesting that health promotion is in a particularly invidious epistemic position. We have a very good knowledge of the natural history of many diseases (tooth decay, for example). So, we can say with relative confidence what would have happened if, for example, one had not visited the dentist and had an extraction. And so we can be relatively confident about the expected utility of such a health care intervention. But behaviour change is far murkier. The causal pattern for behaviours is much less clear. Lots of things influence behaviours. Perhaps the clients would have changed their health behaviours without health promotion activities. Perhaps the health promotion intervention is useless because it addresses the wrong reasons for which people act the way they do. So, epistemologically speaking, health promotion is in a worse position than dental care, vis-à-vis its expected utility. Hence, in a coruscating piece, McCormick (1994) concludes from the lack of conclusive evidence that identifying and modifying risky health behaviours ushers in health gain that '[g]eneral practitioners would do better to encourage people to live lives of modified hedonism, so that they may enjoy, to the full, the only life they are likely to have'.

This brings us to the nub of the problem. Is the benefit to be expected from health promotion activities especially difficult to calculate? The sceptic about health promotion wants us to think so. But perhaps this is too sceptical. For one thing, we should not think of this as an 'all or nothing' thing, i.e., that all health promotion is, or is not, justifiable by reference to expected utility. We can distinguish between health promotion programmes in terms of those that are easier than others to justify by their expected utility. Some behaviours are relatively easy to modify. Some techniques are known to be relatively effective. So, the sceptic is not right to dismiss health promotion interventions *en masse*. Furthermore, there are myriad, perfectly rational ways of calculating the expected utility of behaviour modification programmes. Many of these have not been fully exploited. For example, we might utilize findings from neighbouring fields, including human sciences such as psychology, and economic sciences such as marketing. In sum, a case for the defence of health promotion can be made: justifying health promotion interventions aimed at behaviour modification is, admittedly, a tricky business, but not as hopeless as the sceptic wants us to believe (cf. Buchanan 2000; Whitelaw and Watson 2005).

Ethics and behaviour modification techniques

In order to pursue the ethics of behaviour modification we need to sketch out the main behaviour modification techniques (Callahan 2000). The focus in this section is on State-funded attempts at behaviour change. (Some of the techniques discussed here can be construed as nudges, the strategy for getting people to choose healthily favoured by libertarian paternalists, which was analysed in Chapter 4.)

Mass health communication campaigns

Health communication campaigns comprise the main type of State-funded interventions aimed at changing health behaviours. These include promotional activities such as health education, health information and health advice. Despite appearing innocuous, health communication campaigns raise some disquieting issues (Faden 1987; Gostin 2002a: 345ff; Salmon 1989; Witte 1994; Gostin 2000; Guttman 2000; Guttman and Salmon 2004). They can be stigmatizing (educating the public about AIDS is a well-known example; Douard 1990). More subtly, they can tacitly reinforce social conventions detrimental to sections of society (Saha 2002). Some health communication campaigns are simply patronizing, or otherwise offensive (Davis et al. 1995). They can be used cynically, as, for example, when politicians or the health service want to give the impression that a public health issue is being addressed, whilst knowing that the relevant campaign is unlikely to be effective: 'The sad but plain truth is that a substantial proportion of the population is not interested in messages about their health if these messages prescribe a behavioural change. Health recommendations are mainly embraced by the healthy' (Michels 2005: 3). In some campaigns, health promoters are tempted to indulge in deceptive devices, such as exaggerating the health benefits of behaviour change, downplaying or ignoring detrimental evidence, and using subliminal health messages (Campbell 1990; Johannesen 1996).

Social marketing is an aspect of health communication (Andreasen 2001). Commercial advertising and marketing are very closely allied to what health promoters are attempting in that both aim to motivate behaviours by manipulating preferences. Since commercial advertising and marketing are highly successful industries, it seems natural that health promotion has much to learn from them. However, this idea is troubling:

> By imitating the techniques of the business marketer, who very often appeals to people's strong longing for social and, in particular, sexual success, one can more effectively make people change their lifestyles than by using the methods of traditional education.
> Is this way of operating, in general, unethical then? (Nordenfelt 1995: 191)

It would not be surprising if health professionals dislike the mores of the commercial world. Even very effective social marketing might be dubious. How far are we justified in employing in the health sector the kinds of techniques one derides in a commercial context? How much does the end justify the means: should public money be spent employing an expensive, but effective, private advertising or marketing firm to manipulate people's preferences and choices?

Along similar lines, but more Draconian, is State manipulation of health behaviours by censoring advertising. The obvious example is the ban on tobacco advertising (Bayer et al. 2002). If advertising is construed as a form of speech, censoring advertising amounts to a restriction of one of our cherished rights, namely, the right to free speech. On the other hand, it is easy to generate a clash of rights. We know full well the power of advertising. So, might one say that an autonomous individual has a right to be protected from the insidious effects of (some) commercial advertising? If so, the advertiser's right to free speech is incompatible with the audience's right to protection. If this seems unpersuasive, it can be made more convincing by changing the nature of the audience. Even when restricted, advertising is a blunt tool that influences the preferences and choices of, for example, children as well as adults. Then a stronger version of the clash of rights argument suggests itself: censorship is justified by children's rights to protection from the insidious effects of commercial advertising (Gostin 2000).

Specific interventions

Apart from mass health communication campaigns, health promoters design and implement a very diverse range of specific interventions aimed at modifying discrete health behaviours. For example, the connection between smoking and the health of the foetus is now relatively common knowledge, so health promotion experts design and implement smoking cessation services aimed at pregnant women. Again, such apparently innocuous health promotion activities raise ethical worries. How sound is the empirical basis for the programme? Is it implemented properly or does it waste resources because it is merely 'bolted-on' to other activities? Could the resources it requires evidently have been put to better use? How manipulative is the service: so manipulative as to flout the woman's autonomy? And how far down this road is the medical establishment prepared to travel? For example, would it be permissible to refuse to treat patients whose lifestyle choices exacerbate their conditions and compromise treatments (Underwood et al. 1993; Hastings et al. 2002)?

Most of the health promotion interventions undertaken by specialists are top-down; i.e., they are initiated by professionals rather than invited by clients. One problem with top-down health promoting is that there is not the implicit contract between clients and health promoters that typically exists between patients and curative health care professionals during therapeutic interventions. The client has not asked for a health promotion intervention. As a result, worries arise about the kind and extent of consent gained from intended beneficiaries of top-down health promotion (Guttman and Salmon 2004: 537–8). A related set of worries centres on the apparent lack of a mandate. Top-down health promotion might seem unlikely to succeed precisely because it is imposed from above; if so, it becomes a dubious use of resources. Bottom-up health promoting sounds more palatable, but it is not unproblematic. In reality, how feasible is bottom-up health promotion? For example, what happens when clients identify what they happen to want as opposed to what well-informed health promoters know they need? No matter how subtly, perhaps the health expert will, and even ought to, influence the thinking and judgement of their clients to 'enable' them to choose 'correctly'.

Health promotion includes not only planned and coordinated specific interventions, attempted by specialists, but also what Naidoo and Wills (2000: 127) call 'opportunistic health education': i.e., ad hoc interventions by health professionals. A classic example is that of doctors informing or even cajoling patients about diet, exercise, smoking, and so on, during consultations on other matters. These interventions are often very questionable. For one thing, they are spontaneous, so a patient might or might not receive health advice depending on such arbitrary factors as how busy a doctor is and their mood; yet, if the information is important, perhaps it ought to be given, and given in a more systematic way. Conversely, perhaps such ad hoc interventions are impermissible. The patient did not request health advice; more to the point, the opportunistic nature of the intervention often precludes any proper discussion of the matter, which might result in a very anxious patient who lacks a context in which to pursue the issue.

Personal financial incentives

An interesting and controversial strategy for effecting health behaviour change involves offering people financial incentives. This should not be confused with the similar policy of offering health care professionals financial incentives to achieve a heath care goal (such as payments to medical practices which meet a target for number of patients vaccinated). In the policies under discussion here, members of the public receive the financial incentive, not health care professionals. The basic idea is very straightforward – people get a financial reward for changing their health-related behaviour – but this deceptively simple idea underpins a wide variety of schemes (Marteau et al. 2009).

For one thing, personal financial incentive schemes have been mooted for disparate health issues, ranging from smoking, obesity and healthy eating, mental illness and non-adherence to medication, immunization, screening and testing, drug addiction, and child development. The sorts of incentive also vary widely. Typical schemes offer a straight cash payment for changing health-related behaviour; but even here there is variation in the amount of money offered. For example, in the UK, patients on antipsychotic drugs in East London were reported to be offered £5 to £15 per injection to encourage them to take their medication regularly. Another scheme, aimed at obesity, involved much larger sums: overweight patients in Kent were reported to be offered £70 to lose 15lbs, £160 to lose 30lbs (and keep it off for six months), and £425 to lose 50lbs (and keep it off for six months). In these schemes the incentive is money, but in others the incentive is in the form of cash equivalents. For example, in one scheme pregnant women were offered food vouchers for giving up smoking: £20 worth of vouchers for giving up for one week, a further £40 worth of vouchers for giving up for a month, and a further £40 worth for not smoking for a year. And in an imaginative variation on this, a scheme proposed in Scotland would offer school pupils points for eating healthy school meals, points which they could exchange for items that would benefit Save the Children projects.

Examples so far have been from the UK but there are financial incentive schemes throughout the world. There are plenty of examples from countries with health care systems similar to the UK's, such as financial incentives for Australian parents to get their children vaccinated. Financial incentive schemes have also been set up in non-Western contexts. In a World Bank sponsored trial, for example, young people in Tanzania aged 15 to 30 were offered $45 (£30) if they tested negative for sexually transmitted diseases over three years. And in Mexico, poor families were offered payments as an incentive to make sure that their children attend school regularly and get vaccinated. This illustrates two features of personal financial incentive schemes. First, such schemes are run not only by governments but also by other institutions, including charities. A particularly controversial case is that of the US-based charity 'Project Prevention', which was reported to pay drug addicts to family plan by agreeing to be sterilized or take long-term contraception. Second, financial incentive schemes are often targeted at particularly deprived social groups because that is where the biggest health problems and riskiest health behaviours are found.

There is a theoretical point to mention. Personal financial incentives to improve health are often discussed in the context of the nudge agenda discussed in Chapter 4, but it is unclear whether financial incentives are nudges. It might seem that there is nothing to rule out money as a means of nudging people towards a certain option; for example, giving people a tiny amount of money they do not need for choosing an option might be considered a nudge. But, as mentioned, the size of financial incentives on offer varies, and many schemes are aimed at the poorest social groups for whom the cost of resisting the nudge would be disproportionately high. So, at least some financial incentive schemes would be too attractive to count as mere nudges. And there is a more general theoretical problem. Thaler and Sunstein (2009), the original architects of nudge, divide human thinking into two systems: the 'reflective system', which is rational, self-conscious, deliberative; and the 'automatic system', which is more instinctive, immediate, habitual. Nudges are supposed to by-pass the rational system and appeal to the automatic (this is what makes them seem sinister: we would not even notice many nudges). But financial incentives work by giving people a reason to do something; they change the cost–benefit analysis of various options, so they engage the reflective system (Oliver 2012).

Focusing on more practical matters, do personal financial incentives for health actually work? Getting people to do things by paying them is entirely commonplace, and there is plenty of evidence that personal financial incentives are successful in the health field by, for example, motivating one-off responses, such as attendance at clinics or uptake of vaccinations. The approach has some heavyweight backing; for example, it was recommended in a report by Health England:

> one of the main problems that face both individuals and the government or other agencies tasked with improving the health of those individuals is that *the costs of most unhealthy activities impact in the future, whereas the benefits from them occur in the present*. Policies have to be developed either that bring some of the costs from unhealthy activities (or the benefits from healthy ones) back from the future, or that reduce some of the benefits from unhealthy activities (or reduce the costs of healthy ones) in the present. (Le Grand and Srivastava 2009: ii)

The problem is whether such policies are effective in achieving long-term changes in habits and lifestyles. This is much less clear (Glasziou et al. 2012). For example, whilst financial incentives might well increase attendance at supervised exercise sessions, there is little evidence that they have the sort of long-term impact on people's lifestyles – their general weight management, regular exercise regimes, etc. – that are hoped for in public health:

> financial incentives are effective in encouraging people to perform clearly defined, time-limited, simple behavioural tasks, such as keeping appointments, and also in encouraging participation in lifestyle programmes, but [that] the healthier behaviour is not maintained. Financial incentives are not effective when the behaviour change required is complex, for example, giving up smoking. (Jochelson 2007: 2)

Regarding the ethics of this sort of scheme, Ashcroft (2011) provides a particularly clear and insightful discussion. He structures his analysis by distinguishing the three ethical questions. First, are personal financial incentive schemes coercive? A key point here is that such schemes are often aimed at the poorest and 'offers of even small amounts of money might coerce somebody in poverty' (p. 195). Second, do such schemes amount to bribery? Ashcroft distinguishes two issues here: whether these schemes bribe someone to do something they should not be doing; and whether they bribe someone to do something they should have done anyway. The first issue does not seem relevant because personal financial incentives are offered to get people to do a good thing (i.e., improve their health). But some people worry that overly liberal public health policies allow immoral activities such as underage sex and illicit drug use (a point familiar from the discussion of harm reduction in Chapter 8). For example, if you think underage sex is immoral, you will think paying teenagers to get screened for Chlamydia is wrong (Ashcroft 2011: 194). Regarding the second issue, where is the moral harm in paying someone to do something they should do anyway? Of course, doing so is a waste of money so there is a straightforward resource argument. But there is a more subtle point – one that connects with other issues in medical ethics, such as the objection to a market in donor organs that transplant organs should be given as gifts – namely, that some cases are morally repugnant:

> many parents would think it wrong to pay their child to do their homework, and wrong to pay them to clear Granny's garden of fallen leaves, but acceptable for them to be paid by a healthy adult neighbour. On the other hand, Granny might well give the child a token reward for being a good boy, having tidied her garden, being careful to make it clear that it was a gift, not a payment for work. (Ashcroft 2011: 196)

Ashcroft's third question about the ethics of personal financial incentives is: do they undermine autonomy? Standard schemes surely do not because, as just mentioned, financial inducements engage the 'reflective system', i.e., our rationality, which is the hallmark of autonomy. But there are troubling cases. One example involves offering financial incentives to mentally ill patients to take their medication. The complication here is that the patients' autonomy is already compromised by their condition – hence, in extreme cases, mentally unwell patients lack the capacity to consent – not the financial incentives themselves. Still, it might well be considered dubious to offer money to people, knowing that their ability to rationally deliberate is compromised by mental illness (see also, Halpern et al. 2009; Lunze and Paasche-Orlow 2013).

The healthy environment

Another sort of health promotion intervention involves manipulating the environment with the intention of making healthy choices easier. Health promotion in this sense is very much in line with libertarian paternalism and the 'nudge' agenda, discussed in Chapter 4. There are various, now well-established approaches, such as 'healthy public policy', the supportive environment approach, and community strengthening. For example, a fiscal, transport or education policy might be undertaken neither by health promotion experts nor in the name of health promotion but, nonetheless, be intended to make it more likely that people will choose 'healthily' by manipulating the environment in which they choose. Examples from food policy initiatives include food price restructuring, clearer food labelling, and nutritional standards in schools and other public institutions. Health promotion processes such as 'healthy public policy' generate distinctive worries centring on the legitimacy of State-funded manipulations of our environment. How secure is the State's vision of the way the environment should be? How far is it legitimate for the State to go in influencing the environment? How can the success of doing so, in terms of specific health gain, be evaluated?

One means that the State employs to influence the environment and thereby health behaviours is to remove the means by which one can act on a risky choice. A well-established, and apparently uncontroversial, example is making certain dangerous drugs available only on prescription. This sort of intervention is not a case of 'nudging' people towards healthy behaviour because the unhealthy options are simply unavailable. Problems with this strategy arise when the means to behave riskily have become a familiar part of our landscape, and the State attempts to remove them. An example is the enforced removal from schools of vending machines that sell unhealthy products. It seems much more illiberal to forcibly remove vending machines that have been there for some time, than not to allow them into schools in the first place. Typically, it is met with the liberal objection that the policy violates a right to choose, familiar from Chapter 3.

The State can influence health behaviours via environmental manipulations by allowing the means to act on a risky choice, but making them more expensive. The obvious examples are so-called 'sin taxes' on cigarettes and alcohol. Again, numerous issues are raised by an apparently justifiable practice (Sirico 1995; Lorenzi 2004). One concern introduces the notion of negative externalities. The negative externalities of, for example, smoking include the cost of providing health care to patients with, and lost productivity due to, smoking-related diseases. Perhaps cigarettes can be taxed up to the point at which costs due to negative externalities are recovered. But are negative externalities accurately calculable? If not, is there an element of deception and manipulation here, a masking of the real reason for the heavy tax burden? Besides, it is well known that the burden of sin taxes falls disproportionately on the most vulnerable because it is the least well off members of society who indulge in 'sinful' consumption (Department of Health 1998). Does this make sin taxing inequitable because it limits the consumer choices of poorer people more than the middle classes; conversely, is it vindicated precisely by hitting the real 'sinners' hardest? Sin taxes are sometimes justified by their effect on the next, not the present, generation, who will avoid the influence of growing up around the targeted behaviours. But the more successfully one argues in favour of sin taxing, say, cigarettes, the more pertinent the following question: if a heavy tax on cigarettes is justified, why not a heavy tax on fatty foods? To tax the one but not the other seems inconsistent; but, intuitively, to sin tax certain foods is far more contentious, raising the question as to where sin taxing ought to end (cf. Marshall 2000).

Some of the most prominent, and most frequently discussed, State attempts to change health behaviours comprise straightforward legislative changes. Clear examples include seat belt and motorcycle crash helmet legislation. The question of paternalism is at its most pertinent here. On the one hand, there are many examples of perfectly well-established and accepted paternalistic public health policies (prescription-only medication has already been mentioned). On the other, there is the perennial question as to the extent to which paternalism is justified in the name of population health. These waters are muddied by an issue that becomes prominent in the next section: most of the legislation in question outlaws behaviours that are harmful not only to the agent but also to third parties. For example, the road traffic accident victim whose condition is due to refusing to wear a seat belt places a burden on people around him (notably, his family) and society at large (principally, in the form of health care costs). Can paternalism in the name of public health be justified by saying that it is in the interests of third parties, or is this disingenuous, an excuse for what is in fact paternalistic legislation? Note, too, that legislation creates ethical dilemmas for researchers looking into criminalized health behaviours; for example, Buchanan et al. (2002) describe the ethical dilemmas faced by ethnographic epidemiologists studying the illegal behaviours of injection drug users.

So far, the paradigm has been State-backed interventions to change health behaviours amongst typical members of society. But minority members of society in a position of intransigence raise distinctive issues. Some people are not able to understand health promotion messages, including children, some of the elderly, and some who are learning disabled or mentally ill (Eng et al. 1997). Others are unable to respond to health promotion because they belong to a strong, homogeneous culture that requires certain behaviour patterns; for example, in some minority cultures, there are religious behavioural prescriptions. And other members of society are unable to comply with advice about health behaviours because of 'internal compulsion', notably addiction. What are the ethics of health promotion in such cases of intransigence? Is the health promoter justified in more or less ignoring autonomy, since it is so severely compromised anyway? Is there even greater onus on the health promoter to create and maintain the possibility for autonomy since so many undermining factors are at work? Is it permissible to accept that the behaviours in question will persist, so the best approach – as discussed in Chapter 8 – involves harm reduction strategies aimed at minimizing their detrimental impact (Newcombe 1992; Nordenfelt 1995: 194–6; Elovich 1996)?

Justifying interventions to modify health behaviours

It is clear from the sketch in the previous section that there are numerous, dissimilar ways to manipulate health behaviours that present various ethical issues. How might they be addressed? A professional code of conduct for health promoters such as that published by the Society of Health Education and Health Promotion Specialists (2007) might seem like the place to turn. But as Sindall (2002) – who usefully describes the increased interest in making the ethical aspects of health promotion more explicit – concludes, the discipline as yet lacks a sophisticated intra-professional discourse on ethics. Besides, a professional code of conduct is a good place to start the ethical debate, not a way to avoid the arduous business of proper ethical reflection. Likewise, a number of commentators have applied the four principles of biomedical ethics explained in Chapter 2 (Naidoo and Wills 2000); but, as Cribb and Duncan (2002: 41–3) effectively argue – and very much in keeping with the view of the four principles presented in Chapter 2 – 'the principles are useful up to a point but cannot be applied without many other more specific value judgements being made' (cf. Duncan and Cribb 1996; Sindall 2002: 202).

One might conclude from this that it is best to take a case-by-case approach, i.e., to clarify and discuss the specific details of discrete health behaviour modification techniques and campaigns. There is something right about this because, in the end, the moral merits of specific attempts at behaviour modification have to be examined in their own rights. Nonetheless, for all the variety in ways of modifying health behaviours and the ethical challenges they raise, ethical problems in health promotion all share common roots. For one thing, they all start from the same point:

> While it is generally accepted that each of us is, to a certain extent, 'dangerous to our own health,' there is far less agreement on what can or should be done about making people less foolish. In particular, there is the question of how far government should go in fashioning lifestyles to minimize the physical and mental harm we inflict upon ourselves and others in society through risky personal choices. (Leichter 1991: xiii)

Furthermore, there is a basic dilemma at the heart of the ethics of health promotion as behaviour modification, between a light touch and a heavy hand. On the one hand, if health promoters keep a light touch they thereby fully respect the individual's right to decide how they want to live their lives, but are unlikely to achieve serious health gains by effectively modifying behaviours. On the other hand, if health promotion is heavy-handed then it might well be very effective in curbing risky behaviour and thereby achieve significant public health gain, but only by violating an individual's freedom, autonomy and right to self-determination (Williams 1984). This clash between consequentialist and other considerations is familiar from the discussions in Part I. The main justification for health promotion as behaviour modification is consequentialist: as Nordenfelt (1995: 189) puts it, there is 'a general utilitarian motivation for work towards health', namely, that promoting health behaviour changes will, it is anticipated, produce utility in the form of health gain. But, on the other hand, if one goes too far in pursuit of health gain by promoting behaviour modification, personal liberty, the principle of autonomy and right to self-determination are compromised.

It is worth pausing to point out that the health establishment has always been aware of this central dilemma. To illustrate, consider two quotes from well-known and influential official reports of the 1970s. First, the Lalonde Report – which has already been discussed in this chapter – revealed concerns about 'whether, and to what extent, government can get into the business of modifying human behaviour, even if it does so to improve health' (Lalonde 1974: 36). And, from the USA, the 1979 Surgeon General's report, *Healthy People*, recognized that there would and should be controversy about the role of government in urging citizens to give up pleasurable but damaging habits and lifestyles (US Department of Health, Education, and Welfare 1979).

A good way to pursue our theme is to invoke some concepts and distinctions which count in favour of health promotion interventions. The key is to distinguish empowerment and coercion. Empowerment approaches to health promotion retain a rich sense of the value of personal liberties whilst enabling people to make healthier choices for themselves. This sounds ethically pristine, but it is not always effective. Coercive health promotion imposes certain mandatory health behaviours on people, irrespective of what they would have chosen. This can be justified by appeal to Mill's harm principle, but smacks of paternalism. Let's take each in turn.

Empowerment

To build up a picture of empowerment in health promotion let's start with the notion of voluntary behaviour change (Yeo 1993). Often, health promoters aim to protect and improve health by enabling clients to volunteer to behave more healthily. The distinction between creating and respecting autonomy is important here. We respect someone's autonomy by simply standing back and allowing them to choose and pursue a course of action. For example, we respect a smoker's autonomy by allowing them to smoke. Creating autonomy is more subtle. There are numerous ways of creating autonomy. For example, we create autonomy by informing people of the effects of their behaviours, thereby enabling them to make a proper choice about what to do. Much health promotion involves educating agents about the facts concerning their options. So, for example, health communication campaigns explaining the health hazards of smoking, far from threatening autonomy, help create it. Furthermore, a remarkably large proportion of smokers want very much to give up. Their autonomy is compromised by the addictive nature of cigarettes: their (self-)determination to give up smoking is undermined by their addiction. So, lots of health promotion interventions can be justified by arguing that they enable people to realize their genuine preference to stop smoking.

Closely related to the notion of creating autonomy is the distinction between strong and weak forms of paternalism (Nikku 1997). 'Strong paternalism' occurs when one simply rides roughshod over the wishes of others, i.e., when one treats another like a child. By contrast, the idea behind 'weak paternalism' is the same as that behind creating autonomy: people sometimes behave contrary to their real, or authentic, genuine or basic, preferences. So, weak paternalists impose themselves in ways that accord with the real preferences of others. For example, the smoker's genuine and authentic wishes are for health and longevity. Their desire to smoke is not deep-rooted, but lies at a more shallow level of their preference structure. To stop them smoking is paternalistic because they seem to want to smoke. But stopping them smoking is weak not strong paternalism because it is in accordance with their most basic preferences. The intervention is more a way of correcting for stubbornness and ignorance than requiring unwanted behaviours from others.

Another important, related notion here is that of 'counter-manipulation'. It is easy to assume that people are free to choose how to behave until paternalistic health promoters come along and influence them. But this is naïve because people are already being manipulated in a plethora of ways, ranging from indoctrination during upbringing, peer pressure, advertising and marketing, habituation, and so on, often to the detriment of their health. None of us is entirely free of such influences on the choices and behaviours affecting our health status. This helps justify health promotion because the alternative is not complete freedom to choose one's health behaviours; rather it is a vacuum filled by all the other, often very dubious, influences on one's choices. Given this, health promotion is counter-manipulation, as opposed to manipulation proper; it is one of the myriad forces motivating our health behaviours, but one intended to counteract those forces that motivate unhealthy choices.

Counter-manipulation most clearly applies to health promotion activities such as social marketing (Ling et al. 1992; Grier and Bryant 2005; Andreasen 2001). As discussed in the previous section, one might think that social marketing is a bad thing because it is manipulative. But, arguably, this is to make the mistake of thinking that the alternative to such influential practices as social marketing is complete freedom when, in fact, the alternative is manipulation by commercial marketers. So, arguably, social marketing is counter-manipulation, where the manipulation proper is done by commercial advertisers who influence the public's preferences by motivating a positive perception of unhealthy options. The social marketer is merely levelling the playing field by combating 'illness promotion' with health promotion. This line of thought can then be extended beyond social marketing to justify other health promotion activities. Health promotion is merely countering the myriad influences on our health behaviours of which we are all, to a greater or lesser extent, the victims.

The three notions clarified so far, creating autonomy, weak paternalism and counter-manipulation, run into the notion of empowerment. 'Empowerment' does not refer to a particular approach to health promotion. Rather, it captures a theme running through various approaches, 'which share a concern with the promotion of autonomy and with voluntary rather than involuntary change' (Duncan and Cribb 1996: 340). So, empowerment in health promotion is based on the assumption that voluntary change is better than involuntary change. The aim of health promotion is to support people in making autonomous, voluntary behaviour changes. The health promoter is a facilitator whose objective is to enable the client to choose freely to behave more healthily.

Empowerment approaches in health promotion are laudable because they aim at behaviour change whilst respecting the right to self-determination. But they are also deeply problematic (cf. Duncan and Cribb 1996; Whitelaw and Whitelaw 1996; Coveney 1998). One obvious problem is that empowerment assumes that health promoters know their clients' real preferences better than they do themselves. There is support for the idea. Everyone has experienced coming to realize that they did not really want what they thought they wanted. And people very often assert preferences, not in a thoughtful and principled way, but without having considered the matter much. Furthermore, we can develop criteria for identifying real, as opposed to inauthentic, preferences: for example, my real preferences are those I would arrive at if I were fully informed of the relevant facts, if I had properly reflected on the matter, and if I would be glad to have them fulfilled. Nonetheless, the idea that health promoters know their clients' preferences better than they do themselves remains fundamentally questionable. It is a fact – one that was discussed in Chapter 1 – that health is only one of the things people value, and very often other goods are valued more highly. It is dangerous to simply assume that, since people really prefer health and longevity to anything else, health promotion interventions are justified in the name of empowerment.

Furthermore, even if these initial worries about empowerment approaches can be alleviated, there is a deeper problem. This deeper problem needs to be explained carefully because it is not always well captured. For example, Duncan and Cribb (1996) put it in the following terms: 'Can the two separate intentions – allowing self-determination and seeking health improvement – be reconciled?'; and they ask, 'do advocates of empowerment want to help people or do they want to change people?' (p. 341). But the problem with empowerment is not so much one of reconciliation or clarification. The real problem is that empowerment begs the question. Recall that the dilemma at the heart of the ethics of health promotion is between 'two of our most prized social values, personal freedom and good health' (Leichter 1991: xiii). The idea at the heart of empowerment in health promotion is, let's have both: i.e., let's gain health by modifying behaviours whilst allowing personal freedom. But it is a dilemma. In other words, the two values are incompatible (if they were compatible there would not be a dilemma between them). One cannot respond to a dilemma between A and B by saying, let's have both.

So, arguably, empowerment approaches beg the central ethical question in health promotion.

Coercion

Another set of approaches in health promotion is to make the healthy options mandatory. At this point the distinction between persuasive and coercive health promotion is important (Wikler 1978). Persuasive health promotion invites, but does not require, a health behaviour change. Coercive health promotion does not merely invite, but also requires, certain behaviours by making them mandatory. Generally, the empowerment approaches to health promotion discussed in the previous subsection are persuasive. More specifically, health communication campaigns that inform and advise people about health behaviours – such as diet, exercise and smoking – but do not require behaviour changes, are also persuasive. So, too, are smoking cessation services aimed at pregnant women, intended to get them to see that giving up is in their real interests, but which contain no sanction on continuing to smoke. Many manipulations of the environment are also persuasive: building more cycle lanes, or subsidizing healthy foods, for example, are conducive to, but do not require, healthy choices and behaviours. By contrast, the clearest examples of coercive types of health promotion activities involve legislation: the laws on seat belts and motorcycle crash helmets have already been mentioned; other examples include legislating for health and safety at work, the hygienic disposal of waste, and criminalizing drug use.

There is an immediate complication because this distinction between persuasion and coercion is unclear. There are ambiguous policies: is a policy of refusing to treat smoking-related illnesses persuasive or coercive? And there is vagueness, in the sense that, at the border, it is unclear whether an intervention is persuasive or coercive. For example, a government policy to increase tax on cigarettes by 1 per cent would be persuasive, and a tax increase of 1,000 per cent would be coercive (although smokers would be technically at liberty to buy cigarettes, in fact they are put beyond their financial reach). But there is no bright line, no particular percentage increase, at which a sin tax on cigarettes flips from persuasion to coercion. This vagueness reappears in other ways. A health-promoting law that is properly enforced is coercive, and a health-promoting law that is never enforced is at best persuasive; but there is no bright line at which a law is enforced just enough to be coercive. Also, what is presented as a case of persuasion might in effect be one of coercion: a patient might be 'informed' by a health professional of the health benefits of certain behaviours in a way that makes them feel they have no real choice but to comply with the 'advice':

> Professionals may exert considerable pressure on their clients because they are seen as 'experts' and this can undermine people's freedom to choose ... In providing people with information and support to make an informed decision it is often quite difficult to avoid putting pressure on them to make the 'right' decision. After all, that is what you want them to make! (Katz and Peberdy 1997: 98)

Nonetheless, the point for our purposes is that there is a continuum of behaviour modifications 'from those which are most compatible with autonomous choice and action (persuasion) to those which are least compatible (coercion)' (Tountas et al. 1994: 847; cf. Yeo 1993: 226). At one pole, the client is merely provided with 'information and support to make an informed decision'. We move from that pole along the continuum to more and more coercion until we reach the other pole, at which there are clear cases of coercion.

Interestingly, Mill, the doyen of classical liberalism, seems explicitly to sanction persuasion to influence an individual. The famous harm or liberty principle discussed in Chapter 3 says that 'the only purpose for which power can be rightfully exercised over any member of a civilized community, against his will, is to prevent harm to others. His own good, either physical or moral, is not a sufficient warrant.' But it continues: 'These are good reasons for remonstrating with [any member of a civilized community] or reasoning with him or persuading him or entreating him [but not for] compelling him, or visiting him with any evil in case he do otherwise' (Mill 1975: 15).

Mill clearly thought persuasion was permissible and, intuitively, this seems correct. So, staying at the first pole of the continuum just described, arguably, Mill's harm principle does not apply to clear cases of persuasive health promotion. This is because Mill was concerned with the exercise of power against one's will, and persuasive health promotion leaves the individual at liberty to exercise their will (albeit in the hope that they will exercise it in a particular way). Of course, the further one travels along the continuum to coercion, the less convincing this defence of health promotion becomes. Nonetheless, if we stay with clear cases of persuasive health promotion for a moment, it seems clear that they can escape Mill's liberal sanction.

But the main question to address here is whether it is permissible to coerce people into behaviour change. Mill's harm principle says that power can be exercised against the will of individuals 'to prevent harm to others'. Apparently, the liberal objection does not apply to health promotion that targets health behaviours detrimental not only to oneself but to others too. But there is a general problem as to how to interpret the exemption here. How much health promotion can be justified by reference to third-party harms? There are numerous difficulties here. Take smoking as an example. What counts as a harm? Perhaps there are some fairly straightforward risks to third parties such as the harm done to the foetus by the mother's smoking. But what about smoking in well-aired public places? Does the harm have to be physical, or is aesthetics enough: is it enough that your smoking spoils my meal?

Also, how far can a smoker go in reassuring others that he or she is intent on protecting third parties? Contrast two kinds of smoker. The first smokes very heavily but at no apparent risk to anyone else (they live alone, are not pregnant, never smoke in public, and so on; what Nordenfelt (1995: 193) calls, 'the lonely smoker'). The second smokes very heavily and at great risk to others (they are pregnant, have small children in the house, smoke in confined spaces with others, and so on). The liberal might say that coercive health promotion offends Mill's harm principle only in the first, and not the second, kind of case. But how convincing is this? Even the first of our two smokers burdens society because they expect to get treated for their smoking-related diseases, which takes up general health resources. But is economic harm a real harm? Besides, this cost can be factored out: suppose that the lonely smoker resolves, were they to be diagnosed with a smoking-related illness, to pay for their treatment privately. Are they still burdening society? After all, they live a truncated life (not as healthy, not as long), so they contribute less to the general good than had they not smoked. This is a type of third-party harm, so we can intervene on Mill's principle. But this is starting to seem far-fetched. For one thing, perhaps this person was a better teacher or doctor or whatever because they were happier due to smoking. Even if not, the argument rests on the rather fanciful assumption that we have a duty to be as beneficial to society as possible.

At its most general, the worry here is this. Interventions in the interests of third parties are permissible on Mill's principle. But there is no bright line distinguishing significant and insignificant 'harm to others'. We have to draw the line ourselves. Draw it too narrowly, and we miss out on permissible behaviour modification techniques. Draw it too widely, and we obliterate the distinction between self-directed and other-directed harms (everything causes some very small other-directed harms to society in general, or the economy, or future generations). It is here that the debate between individualism and communitarianism (Chapter 4; cf. Cribb and Duncan 2002: 61–80) is at its most influential in the ethics of health promotion. Roughly, the more individualistically minded one is, the more one will prioritize individual rights over protecting third parties. Hence, the more resistant one will be to coercive health promotion aimed at third-party protection. For example, one will be very reluctant to endorse a ban on smoking in public places. By contrast, the more communitarian one is, the more one will prioritize third-party protection over the exercise of individual liberties, and the more accepting one will be of coercive health promotion that curtails individual rights for the sake of third-party protection. For example, one will be less reluctant to endorse a ban on smoking in public places. To reiterate, this is not a factual matter; rather, having got all the facts in, a value judgement is required that will in large part depend on such things as the extent of one's liberal and communitarian leanings.

Concluding remarks

The aim of this chapter is to explore ethical issues raised by health promotion as behaviour modification. The notion of health behaviour modification was clarified. Two worries about behaviour modification – that it amounts to victim-blaming, and that it is inevitably epistemically insecure – were met. Having described the main behaviour modification techniques and ethical issues raised by them, various grounds for justifying interventions designed to change health behaviours were discussed. This invoked concepts and distinctions such as creating as opposed to respecting autonomy; weak as opposed to strong paternalism; counter-manipulation; persuasive as opposed to coercive health promotion; empowerment; and intervention to modify health behaviours in the interests of third parties. Worries that health promotion as behaviour modification is overly paternalistic can be alleviated by reference to these. Of course, this is not intended as a solution to the problem of health promotion ethics, because quite how best to apply the concepts and distinctions covered in this chapter to specific contentious programmes of modification remains a matter of ongoing debate.

8   Harm Reduction

The previous chapter discussed behaviour modification, i.e., attempts to change how people behave with a view to promoting their health. This chapter is also concerned with people's health behaviour but there is a crucial difference. The techniques discussed in the previous chapter are primarily intended to get people to stop behaving in unhealthy or risky ways; by contrast, this chapter focuses on public health interventions not primarily aimed at getting people to give up their unhealthy or risky behaviour but at reducing the harm associated with such behaviour. Such interventions are referred to generically as 'harm reduction'. First, it is suggested that, though it is very difficult to provide a precise definition of harm, this is not a big problem because it is not hard to describe and illustrate harm reduction strategies. Then the ethically controversial nature of harm reduction is discussed. The most pressing ethical question is whether specific harm reduction programmes are justifiable; here, the distinction between harm reduction approaches to legal versus illicit activities is important. In the last section of the chapter a number of particularly interesting and controversial case studies are juxtaposed, each of which illustrates important considerations to take into account when evaluating harm reduction strategies.

Defining harm reduction

Introducing harm reduction

What is harm reduction? The key is to distinguish two responses to an unhealthy activity or risky health behaviour. One response is to try to get people to stop behaving in that way, i.e., to try to get them to give up the activity in question. Policies with this intention are usually referred to as abstinence policies (another familiar phrase is 'cessation', as in 'smoking cessation services'). The other response is to accept that, for whatever reason, it is unrealistic to expect people to give up the activity in question so it is better to allow it and try to reduce its harmful effects. Policies based on this response are known as 'harm reduction' ('harm minimization' is preferred by some writers).

To illustrate, driving cars is dangerous. There are two responses: first, stop people from driving by banning cars; second, allow people to drive cars but reduce the harmful consequences of this activity by, for example, ensuring that drivers keep to speed limits and wear seat belts, and by getting people to drive less by promoting other forms of transport. The former is an abstinence policy; the latter a harm reduction strategy. Cars are thought to be too beneficial to justify an abstinence policy, so a range of harm reduction interventions are implemented. A more contentious example is prostitution, which also creates health risks. Is it better to try to eradicate prostitution altogether by enforcing a legal ban; or should we accept that there will always be a sex industry and focus on reducing its harmful consequences by, for example, screening prostitutes for sexually transmitted diseases and monitoring clients to better protect sex workers?

Harm reduction is now well established in public health as an approach to lots of forms of risky behaviour. But it is important to acknowledge at the outset the strong association between harm reduction and drugs policies. This connection is due to addiction: abstinence policies aimed at intravenous drug use have proved to be unsuccessful because users are addicted. Furthermore, a harm associated with intravenous drug use is one of the most pressing public health problems of the modern era, namely, the spread of HIV. So the idea developed that it is better to reduce the harmful effects of drugs than to try to eradicate drug use. Strategies for reducing the harms associated with drugs include needle exchange schemes and supervised injection facilities for intravenous drug users, and prescription programmes which supply users either with the drug itself or an alternative substance (Beirness et al. 2008). Such strategies are particularly controversial because the drug use in question is illicit and because there has been a 'war on drugs' dating back to the US response to drug use in the 1970s (Drucker and Clear 1999).

Given that drug-related harm reduction tends to dominate the field, it is important to emphasize that this approach is taken to combat other sorts of risky behaviour. Other activities that have elicited harm reduction strategies include smoking tobacco, drinking alcohol and underage sexual activity of teenagers (Rhodes and Hedrich 2010; Marlatt et al. 2012). It is worth noting that many of these activities, unlike illicit drug use, are legally permitted (Beirness et al. 2008: 6–7). A number of specific case studies are discussed in the second half of this chapter.

Attempts to define harm reduction

The preceding subsection suggests that harm reduction is a fairly straightforward type of policy that is easily illustrated. Nonetheless, attempts to define harm reduction more specifically have generated a sizeable literature. For example, Lenton and Single (1998: 214–15) critique three previous definitions of harm reduction (they focus on illicit drug use – a good example of the point just made that this tends to dominate the field – but the definitions they discuss can apply to programmes addressing other activities). First, a 'narrow definition' defines harm reduction in terms of 'policies and programmes ... to reduce the risks of harm *among people who continue to use drugs*'. Second, a 'broad definition' defines harm reduction as 'any programme and policy aimed at reducing drug-related harm'. Third, 'hard empirical definitions' centre on net gains and losses: 'a given policy or programme ... which display[s] a net gain [is] said to be harm-reducing'. Lenton and Single discuss advantages and disadvantages of these definitions before suggesting their own.

Arguably, there are problems with Lenton and Single's analysis. For example, the third sort of definition – 'hard empirical definitions' – seems to confuse the question as to what sort of policy harm reduction is, with whether it is successful; i.e., to confuse a definition of harm reduction with whether a policy demonstrably reduces harm. Suppose, for example, that a paradigmatic harm reduction policy failed to produce a 'net gain' due, say, to being ineptly implemented; according to this third sort of definition it would no longer count as a harm reduction policy, which seems incorrect. This leaves Lenton and Single's first two definitions. As mentioned, they present various advantages and disadvantages of these, but some seem spurious. For example, they suggest that narrow definitions of harm reduction 'may be less appropriate for nicotine [because] most tobacco strategies are aimed at cessation rather than reduced use' (p. 214). But this is not an objection to the 'narrow definition'; rather, it is simply an implication of the definition that smoking cessation services are not harm reduction strategies.

Lenton and Single's analysis is instructive despite these objections. They are right that the central dilemma is between defining harm reduction too narrowly and too broadly. The dilemma is this. Narrow definitions restrict harm reduction to strategies which allow the risky behaviour to continue but try to reduce its damaging consequences. The good thing about narrow definitions is that they clearly delineate a distinctive set of policies; the bad thing is that they are incoherent because policies they rule out – notably, abstinence policies – also have the effect of reducing harm (getting people to give up a risky activity is an excellent way of avoiding its bad consequences). Broad definitions extend harm reduction to any policy that reduces the harms consequent on risky behaviour. The good thing about broad definitions is that they are coherent (any harm reducing policy is a harm reduction policy); the bad thing is that the definition does not usefully delineate a distinctive range of activities: even straightforward abstinence policies turn out to be harm reduction policies on this definition.

Arguably, this dilemma is unavoidable and re-emerges in every attempt to define harm reduction. Take, for example, Lenton and Single's preferred definition:

A policy, programme or intervention should be called harm reduction if, and only if: (1) the primary goal is the reduction of drug-related harm rather than drug use *per se*; (2) where abstinence-orientated strategies are included, strategies are also included to reduce the harm for those who continue to use drugs; and (3) strategies are included which aim to demonstrate that, on the balance of probabilities, it is likely to result in a net reduction in drug-related harm. (P. 216)

This definition does not seem to be more plausible than the ones Lenton and Single criticize. Familiar problems arise. Like 'hard empirical definitions' discussed above, (3) seems to be more about the likelihood that a policy will succeed than about what sort of policy it is. Condition (1) suffers from the incoherence problem with the 'narrow definition' because the 'primary goal' of an abstinence strategy is also 'the reduction of drug-related harm'. Condition (2) describes a mixed programme that includes both harm reduction and abstinence strategies, which begs – as opposed to answers – the question as to how to distinguish these.

In sum, there are unavoidable difficulties in defining harm reduction. But how big a problem is this? Here we can make a move similar to that in Chapter 7 concerning the definition of health promotion: defining harm reduction is unavoidably difficult but that is not a big problem. As should be clear from the start of this section, the distinction between abstinence and harm reduction is easy to comprehend. Illustrating the distinction in practice is also straightforward: providing drug users with clean syringes is clearly a case of harm reduction; incarcerating users of illicit drugs is clearly an abstinence policy. So it seems sensible to accept that the fact that abstinence policies reduce harms makes definitions unavoidably difficult, eschew definitions, and get on with the important business of ethically evaluating this approach to risky behaviour.

Harm reduction: some complexities

This attempt to diminish the controversy over the definition of harm reduction is not intended to deny that harm reduction is a complex sort of public health strategy. For one thing, harm – obviously a concept central to harm reduction – is complicated: harms of what sort, and to whom, are relevant. There is a considerable philosophical literature on the concept of harm but happily this need not detain us because there is something of a consensus in the harm reduction literature on the relevant harms. The UK Harm Reduction Alliance's (UKHRA) account represents this consensus. They list the relevant types of harms as 'health, social and economic' harms; and they list the relevant victims of these harms as 'individuals, communities and society' (UKHRA 2013). This is a very broad account, which seems appropriate. For example, it allows us to include the reduction of harm to those who indulge in risky behaviour (for example, the drug users themselves) and others (including individuals close to drug users, and their communities). And distinctive sorts of, and victims of, harms can come into and out of focus when the discussion concentrates on specific harm reduction programmes.

Another complexity is due to the sometimes convoluted relationship between harm reduction and abstinence policies. As indicated by Lenton and Single's proposed definition of harm reduction, quoted above, it is not uncommon for programmes to combine harm reduction and abstinence strategies. For example, the same drug rehabilitation centre might provide both a support group for those trying to give up drugs and a safe injecting site for those unable to abstain. Other programmes are complex in a different way. They have what might be dubbed a 'double effect' structure: their intended effect is harm reduction but a foreseeable, and hoped-for, side effect is abstinence. An example often used in the literature is that getting drug users onto a safe injecting site brings them into contact with health care institutions and professionals in ways that might ultimately facilitate their attempting to give up drugs. In keeping with the point of this section, none of these sorts of complexities creates deep conceptual problems; nonetheless, distinguishing and relating harm reduction and abstinence components of a complex programme can be difficult.

The ethics of harm reduction

Despite evidence of public tolerance for policies such as distributing clean needles to drug addicts (Dubé et al. 2009), harm reduction is a very contentious public health strategy. Why is this? Consider a typical statement of the ethical problem with harm reduction:

> The most important ethical concern with harm reduction is related to the 'value-judgment' that it is more important to reduce the harms associated with drug use than it is to reduce or prohibit drug use. The controversial character of this value judgment is amplified because the relevant drugs are illegal. Critics of harm reduction have argued that (1) it encourages drug use, (2) it sends a mixed message, and (3) it fails to get people off of drugs. (Christie et al. 2008: 53)

Christie et al. explain the ethical controversy about harm reduction in terms of the 'value-judgement' that it is better to allow a risky activity to continue, and reduce associated harms, than to try to eradicate the behaviour in question. This is a potentially confusing way of putting the point because the ethical problem with harm reduction is often said to be that it is 'value-neutral' with regard to the activity in question (for example, the harm reduction approach does not pass judgement on drug use). But either way we get to the central ethical point about harm reduction, namely, that it allows the risky behaviour in question to continue. This central ethical issue can be further refined.

Justifying harm reduction: two research questions

First, it is useful to distinguish two research questions about harm reduction. The first is whether the harm reduction approach in general is ethically justified. The second asks whether specific harm reduction policies are ethically justified. The difference between the two questions is one of generality: the first is more general in asking after the justifiability of harm reduction *per se*; the second is more specific and focuses on discrete policies. In an informative discussion, the distinction is nicely captured as follows:

> It is one thing to argue that harm reduction constitutes an ethically legitimate social strategy. It is another to determine which harm reduction strategies are ethically legitimate. (Kleinig 2008: 11)

Both are important but, arguably, the latter of these two issues is the more pressing; in other words, it is more important to ethically evaluate discrete projects than to enquire into the ethics of harm reduction *per se*.

To explain, consider an argument addressed to the first of the two research questions just distinguished. Christie et al. (2008: 52–3) say that the 'primary issue to be investigated is how harm reduction ... can be ethically justified'. Their strategy is to 'focus on the generic philosophical aspects of harm reduction' and 'analyse objections to harm reduction in the light of the ethical theories of John Stuart Mill, Immanuel Kant and Aristotle', i.e., utilitarianism, Kantian deontology, and virtue ethics, respectively. Christie et al. conclude that (i) harm reduction interventions are justified on utilitarian grounds; (ii) Kant's ethics are irrelevant because 'the essence of harm reduction is to appeal to good consequences as a justification for specific actions [whereas on] Kant's view consequences are irrelevant to the morality of actions'; and (iii) 'the virtue of compassion would provide a strong ethical foundation for at least some harm reduction policies, without requiring recourse to Utilitarianism' (p. 56–7).

Christie et al.'s argument is certainly plausible. Advocates of harm reduction can defend the approach by appeal to (i) utilitarianism because the point of harm reduction is to achieve the good consequences of reducing harms associated with intransigent behaviour. They can also appeal to (iii) the virtue of compassion because, compared to harm reduction, abstinence policies seem insensitive to the suffering associated with, in particular, addictive behaviour. And (ii) Kantianism is not an obvious source of justification for harm reduction *per se* because the basis of harm reduction is utilitarian (it is intended to avoid bad consequences). But, although plausible, to demonstrate that advocates can appeal to normative moral theory to justify the harm reduction approach is not particularly informative. And since opponents can also appeal to normative theory to justify their objection to the approach, a stand-off looms. This suggests that what matters is whether particular harm reduction policies, as opposed to the harm reduction approach in general, are ethically justified.

This same line of thought can be traced in the context of political theory. For example, like Christie et al., Fry et al. (2007) ask the question whether the harm reduction approach in general is justifiable. They too find theoretical justification, this time in a political theory, communitarianism, which was discussed in Chapter 4. Again, no doubt they are right that advocates of harm reduction can find political-theoretical support in what they call 'applied communitarian ethics' (cf. Loff 2006). So the problem is not that Fry et al. are wrong in what they say; rather, like Christie et al., this way of addressing the ethics of harm reduction is not particularly informative. And the same stand-off looms: opponents of harm reduction will appeal to other political theory to justify their objections. So, better to focus on whether particular harm reduction strategies are ethically justified, as opposed to demonstrating that there are theoretical justifications for the whole approach.

Harm reduction aimed at legal behaviour

Given that the focus is on discrete harm reduction policies, how might ethical analysis proceed? The key is to distinguish two sorts of harm reduction programmes. First, some harm reduction policies address unhealthy or risky behaviour that is legally permitted. For example, unsafe sex, drinking alcohol and smoking tobacco are risky but – at least, in most places and situations, and when practised by competent, consenting adults – legal activities. Second, other harm reduction interventions address unhealthy or risky behaviour that is illegal. As already mentioned a number of times, the obvious example is illicit drug use, but there are other important cases such as underage sex, and illegal practices which continue to be performed in a subgroup of the population for cultural reasons. This distinction is crucial because, arguably, the ethical controversy around harm reduction is of a different sort when one goes from legal to illegal behaviour.

To explain requires recalling the moral and political theory introduced in Part I. As discussed in Chapter 1, the important consequentialist theory is utilitarianism, which states that the right action – in this case, public health policy – is that which maximizes utility (i.e., well-being, welfare or benefit). The harm reduction approach in general is utilitarian because it aims to maximize utility by avoiding or minimizing the harmful effects of activities there is little prospect of getting people to give up: 'The essence of harm reduction is to appeal to good consequences as a justification for specific actions, e.g., needle exchange and supervising injections' (Christie et al. 2008: 56). This is why utilitarianism provides the motivation, and a strong *prima facie* moral-theoretical justification, for the harm reduction approach in general.

Now let's focus on harm reduction policies aimed at legal behaviour. The basic framework within which to ethically evaluate such policies is provided by utilitarianism. In other words, the first question to ask when ethically evaluating a harm reduction policy aimed at legal behaviour is whether it maximizes utility. Deciding this in particular cases could be very straightforward. For example, it might be perfectly clear that such-and-such a harm reduction intervention aimed at a legal activity will fail to maximize utility because it will be ineffective and expensive to implement. Or it might be that there are quite good prospects of getting people to abstain altogether from the behaviour in question so abstinence policies would be ethically preferable to a harm reduction strategy. But other cases will be more difficult and involve a more complex utilitarian calculation.

For example, as discussed in Chapter 1, the way for the act-utilitarian to avoid naïvety is to build more sophisticated features into their analysis of an intervention. The distinction drawn in Chapter 1 between immediate, short-term benefits, and indirect, longer-term consequences, is a case in point. To illustrate, consider the aspect of harm reduction policies that is obviously contentious, namely, that it allows – even, according to critics, seemingly endorses and encourages – risky behaviour. Suppose a harm reduction intervention produces the immediate, short-term benefits of reducing the incidence of a disease related to the activity in question in the next few years. Still, a critic might argue on act-utilitarian grounds that allowing the behaviour to continue means that children will be exposed to, and hence much more likely to adopt, the activity in question; so harm reduction makes it likely that future generations will suffer from the associated disease. Since the disutility that would result in the long term outweighs the short-term benefits, the policy is unethical.

Similarly, the point was made in Chapter 1 that there is a tendency to restrict utility to matters of health, since this is the relevant field. For example, there is a tendency to think only – or at least primarily – of the health consequences of an intervention, and calculate utility on this basis. But all the types of consequences of an action are relevant to a utilitarian analysis, including, but not restricted to, health consequences. Suppose a particular harm reduction policy has positive health benefits; still, allowing the activity in question might incur negative social and cultural effects which outweigh health benefits. Consider, for example, a harm reduction approach to a very provocative cultural practice; this accrues health benefits in terms of reducing health risks associated with the practice, but such health benefits might be outweighed by the erosion of social cohesion or harmony that results from allowing the practice to continue. Similarly, a non-health-related benefit of harm reduction is that it fosters autonomy by allowing people to pursue their freely chosen activities, whilst minimizing associated risks; utility that accrues from facilitating personal choice has to be built into the utilitarian calculation.

This illustrates how an ethical evaluation of harm reduction aimed at legal behaviour might unfold: will the policy in question maximize utility when its indirect and long-term, and non-health-related, effects are taken into account? This might well require a difficult and complex utilitarian calculation, but the important point for now is theoretical: the basic framework within which to ethically evaluate harm reduction interventions aimed at legal behaviour is utilitarian, the fundamental ethical question being whether the policy in question maximizes utility.

Harm reduction aimed at illegal behaviour

Turning now to harm reduction policies aimed at illegal behaviour, utilitarian calculations are important here too (it will always be important to calculate the utility that accrues from a harm reduction policy because, as stated above, harm reduction has a utilitarian motivation). So the considerations relevant to a utilitarian analysis of harm reduction policies aimed at legal behaviour just outlined are pertinent here as well: one should look to the indirect, longer-term, and non-health-related consequences of interventions aimed at illegal behaviour. But harm reduction programmes aimed at illicit behaviour have distinctive consequences. This is because of the particularly controversial aspect of such harm reduction policies, namely, that they allow – and even seemingly endorse or encourage – criminal behaviour.

Consider, for example, longer-term effects of a harm reduction policy aimed at illegal behaviour: what sort of message does it send to impressionable youngsters about legal strictures? How is respect for the law to be engendered when public health facilitates criminal behaviour? Any health benefits from reducing harms associated with illegal behaviour have to be offset by the detrimental effects – which may well be subtle and hard to perceive or articulate – on the criminal justice system. To illustrate, consider the case of Insite, a safe injection facility in Vancouver's Downtown Eastside district. Insite provides a safer injecting site, including providing users with sterile needles, alcohol swabs, etc., and education about safer injecting and basic health care; on-site nurses supervise injections and counsellors provide therapeutic support. When Canada's federal Conservative government applied to the courts to get Insite closed down, a principal argument of theirs was that to allow Insite to continue operating would undermine the rule of law: 'I turn to the Minister's argument that granting a s. 56 exemption to Insite [i.e., allowing Insite to continue] would undermine the rule of law and that denying an exemption is therefore justified' (Supreme Court of Canada 2011: [140]).

In this case the Supreme Court rejected the argument, commenting that allowing Insite to continue 'has had no negative impact on the legitimate criminal law objectives of the federal government'; but, of course, the result of these more sophisticated utilitarian calculations can go either way. To recall a previous example, advocates point out the subtle positive effect of harm reduction strategies of bringing people who indulge in criminal activities into contact with health care institutions and professionals. Insite's clients, for example, are given health information, have access to health professionals, and so on. If such opportunities motivate clients to pursue abstinence, the overall effect of a harm reduction approach is to uphold the law.

Again, much more could be said about the utilitarian analysis of harm reduction aimed at risky illegal behaviour, but the important point is theoretical: utilitarianism provides a basic framework within which to ethically evaluate harm reduction policies aimed at illicit activities. But further to this there is a quite different source of ethical disquiet about harm reduction aimed at illegal behaviour, one not shared with policies aimed at legal behaviour. To explain this it is important to recall deontology from Chapter 2. The core thought in deontological ethics is that actions are right or wrong by their nature, as opposed to their moral value being determined solely by their consequences. For many people, this precisely captures their moral intuitions about a harm reduction response to illicit behaviour: harm reduction, by its very nature, is an ethically faulty public health response to illegal behaviour, whatever the outcome of – and no matter how sophisticated – the utilitarian calculation. Now we can see why the distinction between harm reduction aimed at legal versus criminal behaviour has been laboured: harm reduction aimed at illegal behaviour provokes a distinctively deontological response, namely, that public health policies that allow criminal activity are wrong by their very nature.

There is a complication. The claim that harm reduction policies aimed at illegal behaviour are wrong in a distinctive way can be put in utilitarian terms. Specifically, it can be put in rule-utilitarian terms. As detailed in Chapter 1, rule-utilitarianism evaluates an action not directly – i.e., not by asking whether it maximizes utility – but indirectly, by asking whether the action is in accordance with rules sanctioned by society because they maximize utility. In the present context, a rule-utilitarian analysis would ask whether the action (the harm reduction policy) is in accordance with utility-maximizing rules (in this case, laws). To illustrate, recall the example above of a harm reduction policy which produces the immediate, short-term benefits of reducing the incidence of a disease related to the behaviour in question in the next few years; a rule-utilitarian would object to the policy despite the utility it accrues because it is not in accordance with a utility-maximizing law.

Although this illustrates how an act-utilitarian and a rule-utilitarian evaluation of the same public health policy can come apart, the more important point for our purposes is that no amount of utilitarian thinking – i.e., no matter how sophisticated the act-utilitarian analysis or the shift to rule-utilitarianism just explained – fully captures the sense that there is something wrong in itself about harm reduction aimed at illicit behaviour. To capture this requires deontology (Wodak 2007). Now the question is, how can we explain this deontological intuition: why is harm reduction aimed at risky illegal behaviour wrong in principle? A straightforward answer is that one ought to respect the law, so harm reduction policies that allow, and even seem to encourage, criminal behaviour are wrong even if they can be shown to be effective in avoiding harmful consequences. But this seems to be a mere stipulation, so it is important to be able to ground this reaction in the moral and political theory of Part I.

First, as explained in Chapter 2, a Kantian way of developing the core thought in deontological ethics – that actions are made right or wrong by their nature, as opposed to by their consequences – appeals to universalizability. According to Kant, actions based on non-universalizable maxims are wrong. In the present case, the actions in question are harm reduction policies. The relevant maxim is, allow criminal behaviour for the sake of public health gains. Such a maxim is non-universalizable. For one thing, the harm reducer does not really want everyone to allow criminal behaviour because there are bound to be occasions on which they would deny this (were they to be victims of criminal activity, for example). So, universalizing the maxim involves a contradiction in the will. For another, it is literally not possible for everyone always to flout the law: if everyone always flouts the law there would be no law (there might be formal legal expressions, such as statutes, but law in a substantive sense would have disappeared). So, universalizing the maxim involves a contradiction in conception.

The deontological intuition that harm reducers should not be allowed to exempt themselves from respect for the law can be grounded in various other ways. Here it is useful to recall the political theory from Part I. Liberals tend to favour harm reduction because it allows people to choose risky behaviour whilst minimizing the harms it causes others (Hathaway 2002). But critics on other parts of the political spectrum see harm reduction differently. For example, libertarians are opposed to harm reduction because, as Wynia puts it, they 'want no pesky regulations hindering their freedom of choice'. But ironically, as Wynia goes on to explain:

> Libertarians are not the primary opponents of harm-reduction programs today. Instead, harm-reduction programs are running into much more vocal, and effective, opposition among a group that is emphatically not libertarian: religious conservatives. (Wynia 2005b: 3)

So harm reduction is seen as intrinsically dubious by disparate critical commentators, and from a variety of theoretical viewpoints.

Other theoretical perspectives

So far the emphasis has been on utilitarianism as a basic framework for ethically analysing harm reduction policies, and the further deontological response to harm reduction aimed at illicit activities. Now other theoretical perspectives discussed in Part I can be invoked. For example, to recall Christie et al., virtue ethics provides ethical justification for harm reduction; in particular, the harm reduction approach expresses the virtue of compassion. This is a good point, but moving to the question as to whether a particular harm reduction programme is ethically justified – as opposed to whether the harm reduction approach in general is ethically defensible – allows other virtues to come to the fore. For example, implementing a particular harm reduction policy might take courage on the part of harm reducers to resist legal strictures and right-wing criticism. Conversely, courage might require that public health retains a commitment to abstinence despite the appeal of a 'softer' harm reduction option.

Another case in point is principlism. Christie et al. (2008: 52) reject what they call the method of ethical analysis 'usually employed in the applied ethics field', namely, the 'four principles' approach, saying that their preferred method 'is more robust than simply referring to abstract principles and then using intuitions to determine which principle is most important'. Principlists would object here that applying normative moral theory also combines abstract principles and intuition so it is no more 'robust' than principlism. But more to the point, as argued in Chapter 2, the problem with the original four principles is not 'robustness'; rather, they are not well suited to public health ethics. Hence, principles better suited to public health have been devised which can be applied in ethically evaluating a harm reduction policy (Upshur 2002). For example, the principle of least restrictive or coercive means counts in favour of a harm reduction approach before imposing more Draconian interventions. And the principle of transparency is important because covert harm reduction programmes are clearly dubious. Sets of principles suited specifically to harm reduction programmes have been suggested. For example, the UK Harm Reduction Alliance (UKHRA) has advocated a set of harm reduction principles which include maintaining an immediate focus on proactively engaging individuals, and balancing costs and benefits in trying to reduce harms.

Harm reduction: some cases

In this section some particular harm reduction policies are juxtaposed. These have been chosen because they are particularly interesting and contentious; also, each case illustrates salient considerations more widely relevant to other harm reduction programmes.

Illicit drug use and groin injecting

Given the prominence of illicit drug use in the harm reduction debate, it seems natural to start with a policy aimed at intravenous drug users. Groin injecting – i.e., injecting the substance into the femoral vein – is currently common and increasingly normalized amongst injecting drug users. There are perceived benefits to the user of groin injecting, including speed and surety of injecting, a more intense 'hit' from the drug, and the fact that the injecting site is hidden; and some sorts of injectors are particularly drawn to groin injecting, notably homeless and crack-heroin 'speedball' injectors. But the practice is intrinsically dangerous because it has a small margin of error – it is not hard to miss the femoral vein – a problem exacerbated by the fact that injectors are often in a state that makes them less adept, such as being intoxicated. Specific harms associated with groin injecting include deep venous thrombosis, accidental arterial injecting, venous ulceration, and infections (Rhodes et al. 2006; Miller et al. 2008).

It is well documented that abstinence policies have proved unsuccessful with this group of clients, which invites a harm reduction approach. Recalling the strategy for ethical evaluation outlined in the previous section, the first question to ask is whether the activity in question is legal. In this case the answer is clear: groin injecting is illegal because the drugs in question are illicit. So the deontological response to harm reduction, explained above, applies to the groin injecting case: policies which facilitate illegal behaviour are by their nature unethical. Still, as explained above, a utilitarian analysis is required, and here we encounter a particularly interesting feature of this case study. Let's focus the discussion on two specific harm reduction policies: first, providing information in the form of 'how to' booklets explaining how to groin inject safely; second, assisting and training groin injectors in finding injecting sites other than the groin, in a clinical context such as an injecting clinic. Are these justified on utilitarian grounds?

There are two types of groin injectors. 'Last resort' groin injectors have already used and exhausted all viable peripheral veins so the groin is their only remaining injecting site. By contrast, 'convenience' groin injectors inject the femoral vein for pragmatic reasons, such as wanting a hidden injecting site (Maliphant and Scott 2005). The two policies play out differently for these two sorts of drug users. Regarding 'last resort' groin injectors, there is no point in helping them to find injecting sites other than the groin so – on the assumption that abstinence is unfeasible – benefit is maximized by providing information on how to groin inject safely. By contrast, it would be most beneficial to get intransigent 'convenience' groin injectors to use a less risky injecting site; so it would be inappropriate to encourage them to groin inject by providing them with information on how to do so safely, and better to assist and train them in finding injecting sites other than the groin. This suggests a general consideration when devising harm reduction strategies: from a utilitarian perspective, benefit will be maximized by devising policies sufficiently fine-grained to reflect relevant differences within a target group (Zador et al. 2008).

Of course, none of this will assuage critics of harm reduction. On the contrary, the critic will see here a clear illustration of a slippery slope argument against harm reduction: helping intravenous drug users to find injecting sites safer than the groin is bad enough, but it is even worse to be helping injectors to groin inject. Such critics will claim that this is only a specific example of the general problem with harm reduction, that once we give up on abstinence, the specific situation of some clients will invite increasingly dubious harm reduction strategies. Better, says the critic, not to step on the slippery slope and insist on abstinence-only policies.

Culturally sanctioned health behaviour: female genital mutilation

Another interesting category of harm reduction strategies is aimed at risky health activities that enjoy strong cultural sanction. A case in point is the range of procedures which alter female genitalia for cultural – primarily, religious – reasons. It is important at the outset of discussion of this sensitive topic to be aware of terminological nuances. Phrases used to refer to the relevant procedures include 'genital cutting' and 'female circumcision', but the more pejorative 'female genital mutilation' (FGM) is used by commentators who want to convey criticism of such practices, and is preferred here. There are various forms of FGM ranging from less to more radical alterations; for example, from partial to total removal of clitoris, labia minora and labia majora (Larson and Okonofua 2002). The procedures in question create numerous short- and long-term mental and physical health risks of various sorts, including psychological distress, haemorrhaging, cysts, ongoing problems with sexual intercourse, and pelvic infection; in the most severe cases, FGM can lead to death. So FGM is a serious public health problem, being a cause of both morbidity and death (Shell-Duncan 2001).

But FGM has proved intractable because of its deep cultural roots; in particular, it is prescribed by religious duty: 'A large factor preventing the eradication of FGM is its importance in the practices of many cultures' (Ruderman 2013: 97). There is an important twist on this intractability. One might expect to enlist women within relevant cultures to attempts to eradicate FGM since they suffer the adverse health consequences; it would be natural, for example, to anticipate the support of mothers who want their daughters to be spared FGM. But studies reveal that women in the relevant communities are themselves in favour of the practice. Various reasons have been suggested for this, from the principled – commitment to religious duty, for example – to the pragmatic, including the disastrous social consequences for a family that holds out against the practice, such as marring a daughter's marriage prospects (Reymond et al. 1997; Mackie 2003). But whatever the rationale, eradicating the practice is made harder when women themselves prioritize the cultural imperative over health consequences.

Because of the failure to eradicate FGM, harm reduction has been mooted as the best response. To focus the discussion, consider the specific policy of promoting what has been termed 'symbolic female circumcision'. This refers to making a small cut on the external genitals, under medical supervision and in hygienic conditions. Is this justifiable? On utilitarian grounds, it would seem so. After all, the point of the policy is to 'fulfill cultural requirements while simultaneously preventing complications and lasting harm to women' (Ruderman 2013: 98; see also Galeotti 2007). This seems to be a 'win–win' solution to the problem of FGM: cultural sensibilities are respected and negative health consequences avoided. But some critics are unconvinced by this or any other policy that falls short of enforcing a ban on FMG. This is not based on the standard argument for enforcing abstinence, namely, that the practice is illegal; rather, their objection is that any form of FMG – no matter how symbolic or hygienic – demonstrates and perpetuates a derogatory attitude towards women and female sexuality. This objection can be theoretically grounded in various ways. A utilitarian grounding is that the indirect and long-term consequences of this attitude are disastrous. A familiar non-consequentialist grounding is that FGM transgresses hard-won women's rights.

This gets us to the heart of the matter: ought Western societies and governments to tolerate a cultural practice that apparently manifests and maintains a derogatory attitude towards women and a hostile attitude towards female sexuality, even if – as in the case of 'symbolic female circumcision' – it is hygienically performed? This is a case study in toleration which cannot be resolved here but there is space to make a few comments. It is important to distinguish two contexts in which FGM is practised, which give rise to two overlapping but somewhat different sets of issues. First, FGM is practised in non-Western societies; here, a central public health question is how Western governments and international health institutions responsible for tackling global health concerns, such as the World Health Organization (WHO), ought to respond. For example, is it appropriate or feasible for governments and global health institutions to impose a ban on the practice? Of concern here is cultural imperialism and the extent to which it is permissible to impose Western values in non-Western contexts. Second, FGM continues to be practised within subgroups of multi-cultural Western populations; here the central question is how Western governments should respond to the continuation of the practice within its citizenry. For example, should legal strictures on FGM be established and, if so, what sort?

These two sets of issues are equally important but it is in keeping with the theme of this book to focus on the latter. One response is that 'Western societies and governments should view harm reduction as a stepping-stone to eventual eradication, not a legitimization of a disempowering tradition' (Ruderman 2013: 103). In other words, harm reduction strategies aimed at FGM are 'holding policies' explicitly intended to reduce harms consequent on risky behaviour until abstinence becomes more feasible: 'an *intermediate* to the ultimate goal of eradication [...] the only viable option *at this time* to limit harm to women and maintain cultural standards' (Ruderman 2013: 98–9 [emphases added]). The idea is that, since it would be implausible – even counter-productive – to try to enforce a ban on culturally sanctioned FGM at present, it is better to reduce associated harms until socio-cultural changes make eradication feasible. For example, harm reduction might be an appropriate interim strategy when it is likely that the cultural subgroup will become more integrated into the majority culture, after which a different, more fruitful dialogue between the majority and minority cultural groups will be possible.

Harm reduction strategies aimed at risky behaviour other than FGM can also be thought of as interim. For example, it could be argued that harm reduction strategies for drug users are 'holding policies' until abstinence becomes more feasible. But there are important dissimilarities between the two cases. In particular, some features of drug use – notably, its addictive qualities – make it implausible that complete abstinence will ever be achieved. By contrast, there is plenty of evidence of harmful culturally sanctioned practices dying out as a result of cultural integration. Nonetheless, the plausibility of this defence of harm reduction strategies for FGM is questionable. For one thing, to what extent do the prospects of eradicating FGM increase as a cultural subgroup becomes more culturally assimilated? After all, there is plenty of evidence of immigrant subgroups becoming increasingly traditional to assert their distinctive cultural identity. For another, there is a fundamental tension between 'holding policies' such as 'symbolic female circumcision' and 'the belief that medicalization counteracts efforts to eliminate the practice' (Shell-Duncan 2001: 1014): the safer FGM becomes, the less of a public health problem it creates and, in turn, motivation to eradicate the practice reduces. Bluntly, there is a danger of ending up with a safe cultural practice at odds with women's rights.

Harm reduction and adolescents' health behaviour

Another case study to which the idea of harm reduction as an inter-mediate policy is relevant involves adolescent behaviour. Risky ado-lescent behaviour is wide ranging and includes legal activities undertaken impetuously – driving recklessly without wearing seat belts, sunbathing without sunscreen, playing sports without the proper safety equipment, and so on – and illegal activities such as underage sex, smoking, drinking alcohol, and experimenting with illicit drugs. All these behaviours are associated with adverse health consequences, such as unintended pregnancies and road traffic accidents, and because of the age of this group they cause physical and mental developmental difficulties. An interesting feature of these risky activities is that they interact. For example, there is a correlation between first sexual inter-course, and use of drugs and alcohol: according to one Canadian report, 'influence of alcohol/drugs' was cited as the reason for having sex for the first time by up to 10 per cent of teenage respondents (Council of Ministers of Education, Canada 2003: 82). Given the prevalence of unprotected sex and sexually transmitted diseases amongst teenagers, this suggests that one sort of risky behaviour (using alcohol and drugs) is a risk factor for another sort (sex).

How plausible are abstinence policies aimed at adolescent behav-iour? Leslie (2008) suggests that 'it is highly unlikely that any interven-tions will eliminate these behaviours from adolescence'. This is worth dwelling on because eradicating risky health behaviour by adolescents is distinctively implausible. For one thing – and without wanting to suggest any grand claims about human nature – such behaviour is age appropriate: risky behaviour is common amongst adolescents because of the nature of this stage of normal human development. In particu-lar, as Leslie puts it, adolescence is characterized by 'experimentation and risk-taking'. Trying to eradicate behaviour based on such features is a bit like trying to eradicate tantrums by toddlers: at odds with the nature of people at that stage in their development. Another feature of adolescence is that young people 'tend to reject authority' so attempts to enforce abstinence are bound to meet with resistance and likely to be counter-productive. Not only is eradication unfeasible, it is to some extent undesirable. Adolescence is the phase in their devel-opment when people try out various personae, develop their own identity, and, as Leslie puts it, 'strive for autonomy in their decision-making'. Adolescents are supposed to 'act out' – to experiment, take risks, reject authority, and so on – in order to achieve the transition from dependent recipients of paternalistic supervision to fully formed autonomous agents.

That abstinence is both distinctly and distinctively unlikely invites a harm reduction approach to risky adolescent behaviour. There is a connection here with the preceding discussion of FGM where it was suggested that harm reduction policies for FGM are 'stepping-stones' to the ultimate goal of eradication: typically, the need to experiment, take risks, reject authority and strive for autonomy diminishes as people mature, so harm reduction is an appropriate interim strategy whilst people grow out of adolescence. But at this point a distinctive feature of harm reduction aimed at adolescent behaviour emerges. There are two ways to achieve harm reduction: first, keep the amount of risky behaviour undertaken constant but reduce its harmful consequences; second, reduce – without aiming to eliminate – the amount of risky behaviour undertaken. The first of these is a standard form of harm reduction but the latter comes to the fore in the case of risky adolescent behaviour.

To illustrate, consider sex in adolescence. The former sort of harm reduction strategy keeps the amount of underage sex constant but reduces its harmful consequences. An example is condom machines in schools, which will not reduce the amount of sex teenagers have – and might even increase it – but will help avoid harmful consequences, such as sexually transmitted diseases and unwanted pregnancies. By contrast, the latter sort of harm reduction strategy aims to reduce the amount of underage sexual activity. For example, numerous policies aimed at delaying first sexual intercourse amongst youngsters are incorporated into sex education programmes. Both sorts of strategies are important, but the latter seem particularly apposite for this client group. This is because adolescence is a period of rapid and dramatic maturation with later adolescents being much more mature than younger adolescents. So, bluntly, the later the better: 'delay in initiation of potentially risky behaviours' (Leslie 2008: 56) is always preferable because the later a young person takes up a risky activity the more likely it is to be genuinely autonomous and the more able they will be to avoid and deal with adverse health risks.

So far the discussion has tended to be in favour of harm reduction policies aimed at risky adolescent behaviour. But there is an important caveat. The focus here has been on risky behaviour characteristic of typical adolescents going through a normal phase in the process of maturation. But some adolescents' risky behaviour is due to much bleaker and more adverse circumstances. Toumbourou et al. (2007:

1394) describe this is as 'escaping distress': 'the most severe and harmful substance use problems are prevalent in an important minority motivated by escaping distress associated with development difficulties occurring from before birth (e.g. exposure to alcohol and drug use during pregnancy) and throughout childhood (e.g. child abuse and neglect)'. Promoting health reduction for this subgroup of adolescents might seem complacent. But accepting both that 'escaping distress' is behaviour of a sort different from that typical of adolescents, and that harm reduction might well not be the most effective approach, does not entail a return to the strategy of enforcing abstinence. The problems experienced by this group are far too serious and deeply entrenched to be responsive to such a strategy; they require a different sort of approach, one that addresses the wider social and economic determinants of such 'distress'.

Mental health and non-adherence to antipsychotics

Taking a harm reduction approach in the mental health field creates other distinctive issues. To focus the discussion, consider the case study of harm reduction policies aimed at non-adherence to antipsychotic medication (Aldridge 2012; Hall 2012). This seems to exhibit all the characteristics of a harm reduction strategy. The behaviour in question is non-adherence, i.e., failing to comply with medical advice by not taking prescribed antipsychotics. This behaviour carries health risks for the psychotic patient, ranging from poorer mental health outcomes to psychotic relapse and even suicide. It also risks harm to health professionals, such as the distress of seeing patients refuse medical advice. The equivalent of abstinence strategies in this case are adherence improvement policies. An example is administering the antipsychotic in 'long-acting injections' which, as the term suggests, are administered less frequently, and are effective for longer, than alternative methods such as an oral preparation. This can be enforced, for example by a Community Treatment Order (CTO) requiring a patient to accept medication in the form of a long-acting injection. But the behaviour in question is intransigent in that patients continue to non-adhere by, for example, relapsing even when subject to a CTO. Hence, a harm reduction approach to non-adherence to antipsychotics has been suggested.

This has given rise to some general principles and guidelines. For example, the UK Harm Reduction Alliance's (UKHRA) harm reduction principles mentioned above – themselves derived from principles devised by Lenton and Single (1998) – have been adapted to the specific case of non-adherence to antipsychotics (Aldridge 2012: 90–1). Some of the resultant principles include pragmatically accepting that 'non-adherence is common and enduring', that '[n]o moral judgment is made either to condemn or to support non-adherence', and that the approach 'neither excludes nor presumes a treatment goal of adherence'. Similarly, the patient case study Aldridge discusses suggests some general guidelines for implementing a harm reduction approach to non-adherence, such as sharing relevant information and other resources, encouraging gradual rather than sudden discontinuation, supporting and monitoring the patient during withdrawal, and making interventions to alleviate psychosocial stress resulting from coming off medication (p. 93).

Arguably, a distinctive feature of this case makes a harm reduction approach questionable. The optimal treatment plan for a psychotic patient is always to some extent doubtful. In particular, there is always some clinical uncertainty as to whether it is in a patient's best interest to prescribe antipsychotics and, if so, which to prescribe (including which admixture of drugs) and how long to stay on them. There are various sources of disquiet. Advocates of talking therapies such as clinical psychology and counselling are generally sceptical about the 'medical model' for psychotic illness epitomized by pharmaceutical interventions such as antipsychotic medication. Even assuming that a pharmaceutical intervention is appropriate, evidence on the effectiveness of antipsychotics is murky. In lots of individual cases, non-adherence to antipsychotic medication turned out to be in the best interest of the patient. And there are trends; for example, non-adherence by particularly intelligent patients tends to bring about the best outcomes. Even if adherence to antipsychotic medication is the patient's best clinical option, there are countervailing considerations: for example, taking antipsychotics establishes that the patient is mentally ill; and there are lots of negative consequences of being labelled mentally ill, including stigmatization and reduced self-belief. And non-adherence as an expression of patient choice is a good in itself, moreover, a good of a sort which is not captured in a narrow medical model.

In sum, which treatment option is in the best interest of the psychotic patient is an unavoidably difficult clinical matter:

> The optimal duration of maintenance antipsychotic treatment in patients who are in remission from first episode psychosis is not known ... there is no simple formula for deciding when to reduce such antipsychotic treatment ... It is considered impossible to predict which patients prescribed maintenance antipsychotics could do without them. (Aldridge 2012: 91)

By contrast, behaviour which typically invites a harm reduction approach has two features, namely, that it is clearly risky but has proved to be intractable; for example, in the paradigmatic case, intravenous drug use clearly carries health risks but attempts to eradicate drug injecting have failed. By contrast, non-adherence to antipsychotic medication does not have the first feature because whether adherence is clinically optimal is always questionable so, in turn, whether non-adherence is risky is always unclear. Regarding the second feature, although non-adherence to antipsychotics is ineradicable, this is not for the sorts of reasons that are standard in the harm reduction literature – for example, because of addiction – but because in a large number of cases it is entirely plausible that non-adherence is the preferable option. Given this, it is questionable as to whether it is appropriate to put non-adherence to antipsychotics in the context of the harm reduction debate. Perhaps the more fruitful way to think about this sort of behaviour is in terms of iterative and shared decision making about the optimal treatment plan for an individual patient. What matters is that psychotic patients and mental health professionals – together with others such as social care workers – devise and revise a treatment plan. Suppose, for example, that the doctor prescribes antipsychotics, which the patient declines; this is not best thought of as an opportunity for harm reduction but as an episode in an ongoing dialogue between patient, doctor and others, as to which is the best course of treatment. Harm reduction is the wrong paradigm for behaviour such as non-adherence to antipsychotics.

Active euthanasia and assisted suicide

Another example of a questionable appeal to harm reduction involves various life-ending practices. In particular, harm reduction has been recommended as a response to the covert practice by doctors and other health professionals (notably nurses) of active voluntary euthanasia (AVE) and physician-assisted suicide (PAS). Both AVE and PAS are life-ending practices which hasten the death of the patient, the difference being that in AVE the doctor kills the patient whereas in PAS the doctor helps the patient to kill themselves by, for example, providing a lethal substance. These activities are covert or 'underground' because in most jurisdictions – with notable well-known exceptions, such as Oregon in the US and the Netherlands in Europe – AVE and PAS are currently illegal. Covert AVE and PAS is risky in various ways and for various agents. Risks for patients include the failure to identify genuine requests for help to die – as opposed to, for example, being motivated by temporary depression – and botched attempts to end a life; risks to health care professionals include the threat of discovery and legal censure.

The equivalent of an abstinence policy for covert AVE and PAS is universal enforcement of legal prohibitions on these practices; but this is said to be implausible because there will always be patients who want to hasten their death, and the private and intimate nature of patient–doctor interactions will always provide opportunities for clandestine AVE and PAS. Hence the suggestion that harm reduction is the better strategy (Magnusson 2004; Smith 2007). One harm reduction policy that has been suggested is to legalize AVE and PAS in order to make these covert practices overt, thereby allowing official guidelines and safeguards to be implemented. The structure of this argument is familiar from other well-known cases, such as prostitution and abortion: underground prostitution and backstreet abortions are unavoidable and dangerous; better to legalize these activities so as to avoid harms by implementing guidelines and safeguards.

But the distinctive feature of this case study is that the ethics of the activities in question are essentially contestable. In other words, whether a doctor's hastening death by AVE or PAS is ethically justifiable is something about which equally reasonable, informed, and decent people disagree. For example, the opponent of AVE and PAS can understand a doctor who compassionately hastens the death of their patient to end suffering; the advocate of AVE and PAS recognizes the moral weight of the objection that a doctor's duty is to preserve life not hasten death. This is why the euthanasia debate is persistent: it is an essentially contestable matter of personal morality. This is not so of health behaviour which standardly invites a harm reduction approach; to recall the paradigmatic case, intravenous drug use is not an essentially contestable ethical matter. This brings into question whether the argument based on 'underground' AVE and PAS is best put in terms of harm reduction. The ethical debate about whether to legalize AVE and PAS is multi-faceted. The fact that these life-ending practices are covertly practised and, moreover, covertly practised in more or less inept ways which create risks, is best thought of as a distinctive consideration in that ethical debate. As mentioned, there is a clear precedent here in the debate about legalizing abortion: one argument in favour of legalizing abortion was that 'backstreet abortions' were common, dangerous and ineradicable, so it would be better to legally permit safe abortions in clinical settings. But this was only one consideration amongst a plethora of arguments about this essentially contestable practice. To cast it as a harm reduction strategy akin to providing safe injection sites to heroin addicts is misleading.

An alternative strategy in response to the current situation regarding covert AVE and PAS is more straightforwardly a case of harm reduction. The thought here is that, since legalizing these practices is very unlikely, guidelines and safeguards should be made unofficially available in order to reduce the harm of covert AVE and PAS:

> for the foreseeable future, PAS/AVE is likely to remain illegal in many countries or jurisdictions. The entrenchment of a policy of prohibition should not, however, rule out strategies to guide, influence and educate those who nevertheless continue to participate in illicit PAS/AVE. When euthanasia is practiced outside of a professional framework, it is particularly important that health carers have the opportunity to calibrate their actions against some minimum set of criteria that would serve as a quality assurance mechanism. A de facto euthanasia protocol is better than none at all. (Magnusson 2004: 492)

This is more straightforwardly a harm reduction strategy. An illegal practice is allowed to continue covertly but in such a way as to reduce associated risks. Of course, there is much more to discuss about this. There are practical issues, such as how guidelines and safeguards are to be implemented. And there are ethical issues, such as whether a harm reduction strategy of this sort is bound to make eventual legalization of AVE and PAS more likely. So there is a plethora of ethical and practical issues; and, of course, the pro-life, anti-euthanasia critic will continue to object to any policy which permits AVE/PAS.

Concluding remarks

One of the aims of this chapter has been to defuse controversy over the definition of harm reduction. Harm reduction is a fairly straightforward approach that is easily described and illustrated, so we do not need to get bogged down trying to define it. On the other hand, the ethics of harm reduction is a complicated matter. Here it has been argued that we need to focus on specific harm reduction strategies, as opposed to asking whether the whole approach is ethical. In particular, the distinction between harm reduction approaches to legal versus illicit activities has been laboured. The moral and political theory from

Part I explains why: all harm reduction programmes should be evaluated by reference to their consequences, but harm reduction aimed at illegal behaviour elicits the distinctively deontological objection that it is wrong in principle. The last part of the chapter juxtaposed some interesting and controversial case studies to draw out some salient considerations that often arise in evaluating harm reduction strategies.

9 Immunization

Primary health prevention aims to prevent the onset of a disease; secondary prevention aims to identify people in an asymptomatic population who have developed risk factors for a disease, or who have the disease in a preclinical stage, with a view to undertaking earlier interventions. This chapter focuses on a major form of primary prevention, namely, immunization. The first section clarifies the topic of this chapter, vaccination ethics. The central dilemma is between allowing vaccinees to choose to opt out of mass immunization programmes, and coercing them to participate. Each of the following three sections responds to this dilemma in terms of, respectively, the harm principle, the duty not to infect others, and free-riding.

Vaccination ethics

There are relatively few clear examples of communicable diseases that have been eradicated by means of mass immunization. Nonetheless, the consensus is that immunization programmes are amongst the most successful public health endeavours. This is because numerous serious communicable diseases have been controlled and contained by mass immunization programmes that succeed in attaining coverage rates sufficient for herd immunity (i.e., sufficient numbers of people in the population are immune from a disease to ensure that all members of that population are immune from that disease). There are good grounds for optimism about the continuation of this kind of successful public health effort. Immunization is an established and familiar feature on the health care landscape, there is considerable public support for, and participation in, a variety of vaccination programmes, and new and improved vaccines are being developed to combat infectious diseases. Of course, there are ongoing practical issues about vaccination; nonetheless, mass immunization against infectious diseases seems set fair to continue as one of public health's success stories (Smith 2000).

Dissent

Given their success, why are mass immunization programmes said to be ethically problematic? We can work into this by thinking about why people refuse vaccines. There is now a considerable and impressive literature elucidating dissent from mass immunization programmes. Facts about dissension have been clarified (Smith et al. 2004), kinds of dissent distinguished (Stone 1995), reasons for refusing a vaccine have been delineated and debated (Rogers et al. 1995; Silverman et al. 2002; Calandrillo 2004; Salmon et al. 2005; Lyren and Leonard 2006), and responses to the phenomenon reviewed and advocated (King 1999; Shefer et al. 1999; Szilagyi et al. 2002; Diekema and the Committee on Bioethics 2005). Some authors take a historical perspective, reporting and interpreting past anti-vaccination activities in ways that shed light on current dissension (Nelson and Rogers 1992; Plotkin and Plotkin 1994). Some have taken a social scientific approach, resulting in a sociological critique that insists on properly contextualizing vaccination resistance (Streefland 2001; Vernon 2003). Others combine the two (Greenough 1995). The influence on vaccination decisions of the way relevant information – notably, concerning risks – is communicated to, and perceived by, the public has been discussed (Bellaby 2003; Hobson-West 2003; May 2005). Salmon et al. (1999) take a slightly different perspective by quantifying the risk of taking up the opportunity offered in the USA to be exempted from vaccination on medical, religious and philosophical grounds. Lurking behind this is the theme of dissension and false belief, i.e., refusing vaccinations because of misperceptions, as opposed to true beliefs, about risks and harms (Gellin 2005; Kennedy et al. 2005; Sorell 2007).

No doubt there is unjustifiable dissent from mass immunization programmes, some of which figures later in this discussion. Some vaccines are safe but believed to be dangerous. Bandwagons of ungrounded anxiety about a programme get rolling. Some refusals are not really cases of dissent at all, such as when a parent fails out of sheer laziness or irresponsibility to protect their child and others by a very safe and effective vaccination. Nonetheless, the important point for our purposes is that the history of vaccination makes the following entirely plausible:

> We reach a much harder moral dilemma, of course, in the situation where vaccination may pose a net risk to the individual child, even though a mass immunization policy controls the disease better in the population. In that case we must simply have a clash between the parental ethic of loyalty to one's own children ... and the public need to minimize disease among children at large. (Menzel 1995: 114)

In other words, no matter how many perfectly – or, at least, acceptably – safe and effective vaccines there are, and no matter how much dissension is unwarranted or due to poor communication, there is a central core of cases of dissension that is apparently justified by the refusers' perception of risks and harms associated with the vaccine in question.

The problem central to the ethics of immunization arises here. In cases of less than perfectly safe and effective vaccines, is getting vaccinated a matter of one's own personal or individual choice, or is it right to require or mandate individuals to participate in an immunization programme for the sake of the communal benefit of herd immunity? Are individuals at liberty to refuse a vaccination because it is dangerous, or is this selfish given the public benefits of mass immunization? Is the State within its rights to make mass immunization compulsory or mandatory in order to protect the public health, or is this an excessive use of State power? When implementing mass immunization campaigns, where is the right point to be on the continuum from voluntary to compulsory participation (Gostin 2000: 179ff.; Pywell 2000; British Medical Association 2003; Krantz et al. 2004)?

A familiar case in point is the controversy over childhood vaccinations. Do parents have the right to decide whether their child is vaccinated, or is the State within its rights to make participation in mass childhood vaccination programmes compulsory (Noah 1987; Diekema and Marcuse 1998; Bradley 2000; McIntyre et al. 2003; Isaacs et al. 2004)? That this is highly controversial is clear from the disparities between policies implemented in otherwise similar health care systems. For example, in some countries, the decision is entirely voluntary; in other countries, more aggressive means to ensure the uptake of vaccination are used, ranging from measures designed to motivate people to participate in immunization programmes, to making school enrolment conditional on proof of the child's vaccination status (Dare 1998). The contentiousness of the issue is also clear from specific disputes that fan the flames of controversy, such as the debate sparked by the putative links between the measles, mumps and rubella (MMR) vaccine and risk of autism, and reports of the return of relatively rare childhood diseases because of the numbers of people dissenting from mass immunization programmes (Heller et al. 2001; Morgan et al. 2003; Largent 2012).

Two perspectives

In addressing this problem, two related perspectives must be clearly distinguished and kept in mind throughout the discussion. On the one hand, there is the perspective of the State. From this point of view, the central question is whether compulsory vaccination is a morally permissible use of State powers. Suppose, for example, that there are good moral arguments for allowing the State to impose effective but dangerous vaccines on people; this would provide strong support for policies of compulsory vaccination. On the other hand, there is the perspective of the individual. From this point of view, the central question is about the right ethical stance for an individual to take on getting vaccinated against an infectious disease. Suppose, for example, that there are good moral arguments to the conclusion that individuals have a duty to get themselves vaccinated; this would obligate individuals to participate in mass immunization programmes. These two perspectives are intimately connected: for example, a duty on individuals to get vaccinated would provide support for policies of compulsory vaccination, because such policies could be put in terms of the State ensuring that people fulfil an independently established personal obligation.

There are a number of interesting and important arguments for and against the various State policies of compulsory vaccination, and for and against a duty on individuals to get themselves vaccinated. In this chapter there is time to discuss three of them. This is neither exhaustive – there are other interesting perspectives on the problem that cannot be considered here (Dawson 2004, 2007) – nor conclusive. Nonetheless, the main aim is to pursue the ethics of mass immunization by considering three important arguments. The first is an argument to the conclusion that the State is within its rights to coerce people to participate in mass immunization campaigns.

Liberalism and the harm principle

Viewing the problematic from the perspective of the State, the central question is whether to endorse State-backed policies of compulsory immunization. Such policies represent an interference in individual liberties because someone who wants to dissent from a mass immunization programme is coerced to participate by the State. Immediately, this puts one in mind of the central liberal tenet, the harm principle, first discussed in Chapter 3: 'the only purpose for which power can be rightfully exercised over any member of a civilized community, against his will, is to prevent harm to others. His own good, either physical or moral, is not a sufficient warrant' (Mill 1975: 15).

A simple argument suggests itself: voluntary non-immunization threatens to harm others; the State is within its rights to coerce people against their will in order to avoid third-party harms; therefore, State-backed policies of compulsory immunization are justified. Let's call this the liberal argument for compulsory immunization:

> Infectious disease regulations targeted toward individuals who pose risks of tangible and immediate harm to others ... are well within traditional liberal understandings of the legitimate role of the state. Consequently, liberals would be expected to support liberty-limiting infectious disease control measures (e.g., vaccination, physical examination, treatment, and quarantine), at least in high-risk circumstances. (Gostin 2003: 1148. Cf. Häyry and Häyry 1989: 44; Dare 1998: 138ff.)

Evaluating the liberal argument: three complications

How strong is the liberty argument? It turns on the claim that non-immunizers harm others. In order to evaluate this claim, we need to address three complications. The first complication is that non-immunizers do not threaten or cause harm because, in this case, any harm is due to the disease, not to people's decisions and actions (Dare 1998: 138). This fails to distinguish kinds of harms. One kind of harm agents can cause is in the form of the suffering of actual physical ill effects. Another is in the form of significantly increased risk of the suffering of actual physical ill effects. Contrast, for example, the harm I cause by bashing you in the face, and the harm I cause by tricking you into saying something to someone whom I expect to respond by bashing you in the face. I created third-party harms in both cases: physical pain in the first, and significantly increased risk of physical pain in the second. *Prima facie*, dissenters from mass immunization programmes cause harm to third parties of the latter kind, i.e., significantly increased risk of suffering the ill effects of acquiring a vaccine-preventable disease. Since the State very frequently interferes to coerce individuals to avoid threatening third parties with the harm of increased risks in other contexts, arguably it is justified in making participation in mass immunization programmes compulsory.

A second complication is that one might think that this putative third-party harm of increased risk is morally negligible because it is run only by people who have consented to it. The idea here is that the people who are made more likely to acquire a disease by the dissenters' decision to refuse a vaccine are themselves unvaccinated (otherwise, the vaccine would protect them from the disease). Since they have volunteered not to get vaccinated, victims of the decision not to participate in a mass immunization programme consented to the increased risk. But, as many commentators have pointed out, this is unrealistic (Häyry and Häyry 1989: 44; Dare 1998: 140–1). Generally, the problem is that very many unvaccinated people are unable to choose their vaccination status. Some people have thought long and hard about it, but are ruled out of a mass immunization programme on medical grounds. Others have not provided voluntary, informed consent to remain unvaccinated; rather, the programme has not been made fully available to them, either in the sense that they have not been sufficiently clearly informed about their options, or because of more practical problems, such as the timing and location of vaccination clinics. Also, this is one of the many places in this chapter to bear in mind the general point that, typically, vaccination decisions are made by parents on behalf of children who are, by definition, incompetent to consent.

The third complication is not so straightforward, but is telling in terms of the strength of the liberty argument. The issue here is whether refusing a vaccine is a matter of harming others or simply not benefiting them. This is crucial because the main point of the harm principle is to legitimate State interference in order to prevent harms to third parties, not in order to provide benefits. Dare (1998: 138–40) has an interesting discussion of this, based on Feinberg (1984). Dare points out that it is natural to think of harms and benefits in terms of a metaphor: we harm someone by taking them below a baseline, and benefit them by taking them above it. But there are two ways of describing the relevant welfare baseline: (a) the position the person was in prior to the intervention; (b) the person's normal position. According to (a), we benefit someone by making them better off than they were just prior to the intervention, and harm them by making them worse off than that. According to (b), we benefit someone by making them better off than they normally are, and harm them by making them worse off than that.

Dare makes two moves. First, he suggests that (b) is a better account of the welfare baseline than (a). Suppose a child is drowning and I decline to save him even though doing so would have incurred no cost or risk to myself. Intuitively, we feel that this is morally wrong, and that the State would be within its rights to coerce me to save the child. But this intuition conflicts with the interpretation of harm and benefit based on (a) because, according to (a), I have not made the child any worse off than he was just prior to my intervention. In turn, since I have not harmed him, the State should not coerce me to act. By contrast, the interpretation of harm and benefit based on (b) chimes with our intuitions: to save the child is not to confer a benefit on him but, rather, to move him back to the baseline, i.e., his normal position. Since, arguably, not to do this is to harm him, the State is within its rights to coerce me to do so. The second move Dare makes is to say that the welfare baseline of citizens of the countries he is discussing – principally, Australia and the USA – is informed by well-established, successful mass immunization programmes. In other words, herd immunity to certain diseases is part of the normal position of citizens of such countries.

Putting all this together, to voluntarily non-immunize is to take people in such countries below their welfare baseline – i.e., their normal position, as influenced by successful vaccination programmes – and, as such, is harmful. In turn, the State is within its rights to coerce people to participate in order to avoid such third-party harms. The upshot is that the liberty argument seems strong: it is legitimate for the State to coerce individuals against their will by forcing them to get vaccinated in order to avoid third-party harm. Of course, anti-liberal political philosophies such as communitarianism bolster this. From the communitarian perspective, as discussed in Chapter 4, liberalism overstates the value of personal autonomy and individual freedoms, at the expense of duties and obligations to communities of which we are unavoidably a part. The conclusion that we ought to participate in mass immunization programmes, and that, in turn, the State is not overreaching its mandate by coercing us to do so, is not surprising to a communitarian.

Let's grant for the moment that the liberty argument is as has been suggested thus far. It follows that the State can rightfully impose on dissenters to compel them to participate in mass immunization programmes, even against their will. But this would not justify just any immunization policy, no matter how Draconian. Dare (p. 142–3) makes the point that '[t]he harm principle is usually taken to license only such interference with liberty as is necessary to avert threatened harm'; hence, even if the harm principle endorses State coercion to protect third parties, it is within the spirit of liberalism to prefer the least intrusive forms of coercion. Dare concludes that the New Zealand immunization policy of requiring evidence of immunization *status* upon school enrolment is preferable to the American policy of requiring evidence of immunization upon school enrolment: the two policies are equally effective in avoiding third-party harms, but the former represents less intrusion into individual lives than does the latter.

This preference for least intrusion is a well-established theme in public health ethics and has been mentioned a number of times in this book. One occurrence was in the discussion of principlism in Chapter 2: one of the principles adapted to public health ethics is Upshur's principle of least restrictive or coercive means. Similarly, one of Childress et al.'s (2002) five justificatory conditions 'to help determine whether promoting public health warrants overriding such values as individual liberty or justice' – also cited in Chapter 2 – is that of 'least infringement'. A very clear application of the principle to immunization ethics is by Verweij and Dawson (2004), who recently proposed seven principles for collective vaccination programmes, one of which is: 'Participation should, generally, be voluntary unless compulsory vaccination is essential to prevent a concrete serious harm' (p. 3123).

Two rejoinders to the liberal argument

The upshot of the discussion so far is that the State is within its rights to implement policies that compel people in the least Draconian way to participate in mass immunization programmes. But this is not the end of the matter. The liberal argument is vulnerable to at least two kinds of rejoinder. The first reconsiders the claim that the dissenter harms anyone. Suppose I refuse a vaccination. The central question is, how, and to what extent, have I harmed anyone? The obvious complication here is that, typically, I have refused a vaccine on behalf of my child. This seems like an unavoidably clear case of third-party harm because I have put my child at risk of a vaccine-preventable disease. But, though the conclusion cannot be avoided, it can be counteracted. We endorse parental rights over children, and baulk at State interference in the way individual parents bring up their children, to an astonishing extent. This is grounded in a strong sense of parental autonomy and authority, and scepticism about how successful public agencies would be in usurping parents: 'The default assumption is that parents are the most appropriate decision makers because they know their children well and are in the ideal position to decide what is in the child's best interest' (Lyren and Leonard 2006: 402). Given this, arguably, so far as the parental decision to dissent from a childhood vaccination is concerned, the upshot is a stand-off between two equally powerful considerations. On the one hand, the State is within its rights to coerce parents because their decision threatens third parties; on the other, health-related decisions such as whether to get vaccinated are, traditionally and defensibly, the sole responsibility of parents.

Stand-offs are obviously unsatisfactory, so it is worth pressing on to see what other arguments there are for and against State coercion. One line of enquiry reconsiders just how harmful the decision to refuse vaccination is. Consider two thought experiments to test out our intuitions about this. In the first, mass immunization has almost succeeded in eradicating a disease that requires a human host by vaccinating the whole population. But one person decides to refuse the vaccine, thereby saving the virus by providing a last host. In the second thought experiment, herd immunity against a disease is about to be achieved by vaccinating 90 per cent of the population. But someone decides to replace the vaccine in the stock piles of phials with a harmless but completely ineffective placebo. These are clear cases of a person harming third parties by their vaccination decisions. Niceties about whether the disease is eradicable or non-eradicable, acts and omissions, actual versus risks of harm, and so on, simply go by the board. The State is well within its rights to interfere with the liberty of the agents in these thought experiments to avoid third-party harms.

But now come back to the actual world. Real-world dissension of the kind described in the previous section seems very far removed from the clearly dubious actions in the thought experiments. Numerous factors are relevant here. The agents in the thought experiments are being malicious, whereas the vast majority of voluntary non-immunizers are not. There are no considerations that count in favour of the agents' actions in the thought experiments; by contrast, many actual dissenters are acting on principled grounds. The effects of the imaginary agents' actions are very predictable (the survival of an eradicable disease, the loss of herd immunity), whereas the effect of an actual dissenter's refusal is much less predictable (they, their child, and others, might, or might not, get ill). In the thought experiments, the agents' actions will have predictable consequences whatever other people decide; but in many cases of actual dissension, whether voluntary non-immunization causes harm depends on the decisions and actions of others (for example, herd immunity to an ineradicable disease might well be achieved despite some dissension because large numbers of other people choose to vaccinate).

The point of the thought experiments is to query the claim that real-world vaccination refusals perpetrate third-party harms by setting up a contrast with very clear-cut cases. However, this is inconclusive, and the debate can be continued. Proponents of coercive vaccination policies can complain that, though the agents in the thought experiments perpetrate third-party harms more obviously than do actual dissenters, State interference in the decisions of both are legitimate. Opponents of coercive vaccination can retort that the harm to others perpetrated by dissension is simply too nebulous to warrant anything as Draconian as coercion to immunize. Proponents can respond by saying that a harm is a harm even if it is nebulous in the sense that the identities of the victims are unknown. Opponents can point to other cases of allowing people to make up their own mind in ways that might or might not cause ill-defined harms to unidentified others, and argue for consistency. And so the dispute continues to unfold.

Inconclusive though this is, enough has been said to query any easy application of the harm principle to immunization ethics. Let's leave this discussion with one last, rather subtle, point. This refers us back to the well-spring of liberalism, i.e., autonomy. Recall from Chapter 3 that the liberal tradition in political philosophy is grounded in the recognition of the autonomy of individuals. That is what makes the liberal concession to State interference in individual autonomy so liberal: only harm to third parties clearly legitimizes it. Now, let's reconstruct an ideal case of vaccine refusal. An intelligent, well-informed, competent agent thinks long and hard about a vaccine and arrives at thoughtful and sincere objections. What makes this scenario plausible is the nature of mass immunization. For example, the iatrogenic effects of vaccines are unclear. The success of programmes is questionable. The nature of the harms and benefits is contestable. Facts and phenomenology come apart. Parental imaginings about damaging their child by having them vaccinated are nightmarish. Now suppose that this ideal dissenter is coerced by the State to participate in the mass immunization programme in question in order to avoid third-party harms. This seems paradoxical. On the one hand, coercion is justified by the harm principle. But, on the other, the well-spring of liberalism in general, and the harm principle in particular, is individual autonomy, and our ideal dissenter sounds like a liberal hero, i.e., someone who has, has utilized, and is about to express, their autonomy. So, the liberal is in a quandary between recognizing this admirable expression of autonomy and invoking the harm principle. Again, we end up in an inconclusive place. But, again, enough has been said to query the easy application of liberalism's harm principle to immunization ethics. Let's try another tack.

The duty not to infect others

A second argument to be considered goes as follows. We are creatures capable of infecting one another. This is a contingent fact because, presumably, we might have evolved differently, so that we can neither acquire nor communicate infection. But in the actual world each of us can, and often does, infect other people. This raises a moral question about how one ought to act, or what one should do, given this potential to communicate diseases. This is a very familiar practical matter: for example, parents teach their children that they should cover their mouths and noses when coughing and sneezing, and colleagues castigate one another for coming to work and spreading germs around. Also, there are more serious, high profile cases of relevant behaviours that are downright unethical and even illegal, such as when an individual is convicted of deliberately infecting someone with HIV. This raises an intriguing question as to how to clarify the details of our moral obligations and duties around infecting others.

The strong general duty thesis

Harris and Holm (1995) argue that there is a strong general duty not to infect others. They begin by asking whether there is 'a general duty not to spread contagion' (1995: 1215). Although they recognize that the question arises most obviously in the context of HIV and AIDS, they explicitly widen the discussion to include other contagious diseases, including influenza, and even less serious ones such as the common cold. They claim that the general duty not to spread contagion applies to trivial diseases, and that it is unaffected by the mode of transmission (sex, kissing, working side by side, etc.). They also introduce what they call the 'reciprocity thesis', i.e., that it is only reasonable to expect people to meet the specific obligations this duty places on them – such as staying off work because of being knowingly infectious – if society reciprocates in the form of protection and compensation. (This recalls Upshur's (2002: 102) reciprocity principle, discussed in Chapter 2, that 'society must be prepared to facilitate individuals and communities in their efforts to discharge their duties'.)

In sum, according to Harris and Holm, if I have a cold then I have a moral obligation to stay off work, and the State has a reciprocal obligation to compensate me for any personal costs of doing so – such as loss of income – all because of a duty not to infect others. This thesis puts serious moral pressure on each of us to take every precaution to avoid getting infected in the first place. After all, the best way to avoid infecting others is not be infectious; so, if we are serious about our duty not to infect others, we ought to do everything we can not to acquire communicable diseases. Specifically, and crucially for present purposes, one way of avoiding becoming contagious is to get vaccinated against communicable diseases. So, the upshot is a strong moral obligation to participate in immunization programmes. In turn, if this argument is sound, there are moral grounds for State policies of compulsory vaccination. Far from being Draconian, in enforcing such policies the State is ensuring that people fulfil their moral obligations.

Before evaluating it, it is worth clarifying the relationship between this argument and the one in the previous section that was based on liberalism's harm principle. They are close bedfellows and might be confused. Both arguments, if successful, would justify coercive State immunization policies. And both appeal, centrally, to the thought that dissension threatens to result in the spread of infection. But the argument in the previous section says that such a threat is a third-party harm, and the State is within its rights to compel people to avoid these. By contrast, the idea central to the present argument is that the moral obligation to get vaccinated is grounded in a general duty not to infect others, and the State is within its rights to compel people to meet their moral obligations. This is one of those points at which the distinction between the two perspectives described at the start of this chapter – that of the State, and that of the individual – is useful: the previous discussion looks at the issue from the perspective of the State, asking whether interference is justified; this one looks at the issue from the perspective of the individual, asking after their moral obligations.

Objections to the strong general duty thesis

The suggestion under consideration is that one ought to be vaccinated against communicable diseases as part of a strong general duty not to infect others (Verweij 2005: 325–6). In evaluating this, an objection needs to be dealt with immediately because it is appealing but unsuccessful.

The objection is based on the distinction between acts and omissions. The point of the distinction is that acts are worse than omissions. Compare two scenarios. In the first, someone acts so as to create an evil; in the second, someone creates the same evil, not by acting, but by omitting to act in a way that would have prevented it. For example, compare someone pushing their victim into a river to drown them, and someone refusing to save the drowning victim. Intuitively, we feel that the former is morally worse than the latter. This intuition has proved remarkably influential in various spheres, including the law (sins of commission are punished more heavily than sins of omission), philosophy (the distinction connects with a number of distinctions in moral theory, such as positive versus negative duties), and practical ethics in general and medical ethics and practice in particular (most notably, it underpins the endorsement of passive, but not active, euthanasia).

Now, one can infect others both by acting to do so and as a result of omitting to act. For example, I can infect you with a cold by spitting in your drink, and by not taking the medicine that would have cleared up my cold before we went out for a drink. Is the evil we bring about when we infect others by not getting vaccinated a result of action or omission? Clearly, it is the result of an omission, i.e., omitting to get vaccinated. So – goes the objection – if acts are worse than omissions, then infecting others by refusing vaccinations is not so serious. But this is a red herring for the following reason. Suppose we accept that acts are morally worse than omissions (many people would not: see Tooley 1980). All this proves is that infecting others by acting is worse than infecting others by omitting to act. But it does not follow that infecting others by omitting to act is morally permissible, or anything less than the dereliction of a moral duty. Both can be bad even if one is worse than the other. In other words, it could be the case that both acting to infect others, and infecting others by omitting to act, are cases of failing to meet our moral obligations, even if the former is worse than the latter. The upshot is that, even if we grant the acts/omissions distinction, it does not count against the view that the duty not to infect others entails that one ought to get vaccinated (Verweij 2005: 327).

The better way to evaluate the argument focuses on the basic claim that we have a duty not to infect others. It seems to lead to counterintuitive conclusions. A case in point recalls Harris and Holm's reciprocity thesis, reported above. The thesis is that the State ought to compensate people for the costs of meeting the obligation not to risk infecting others. It is grounded in the idea that it would be unfair to expect people to lose out by meeting their obligations not to spread diseases. But the policy of reciprocation is highly questionable. For one thing, it is not at all clear that it is a duty of the State to compensate people for avoiding the transmission of infections. But, more to the point, even if it were, this is an entirely unworkable policy, practically speaking. To mention just one problem, the onset of diseases is not a very neat affair. Diseases tend to gestate during an asymptomatic period, sometimes taking hold, other times not, and very different diseases share early symptoms. Are we really expecting the State to pay compensation to a worker who thought they might be 'coming down' with something, but in the end were fine? Most obviously of all, the policy is open to abuse.

However, this is inconclusive because it could be argued that the problem is not with the strong general duty, but Harris and Holm's reciprocity thesis. One might endorse the duty but give up the reciprocity thesis. But here a stronger version of the same kind of objection emerges, based on the over-demandingness problem mentioned in Chapter 1. As Verweij (2005: 326) puts it, a duty not to infect others leads to the absurd conclusion that 'morality would ... paralyse us or make us obsessed with all possible (even remote risks of) harm'. Interestingly, Verweij goes on to argue that this is less of a challenge to utilitarianism than to an alternative moral theory, namely, contractualism, which is not central to our concerns in this chapter. The more important point for our purposes is that a strong general moral duty not to infect others entails that we are all, all the time, morally responsible for not putting others at risk of infection; and this is so absurd as to imply that there was not this strong general moral duty in the first place. This seems fatal to the view that there is a duty to avoid spreading contagion.

Now we are in a quandary. On the one hand, the over-demandingness argument suggests that there is not a duty not to infect others. On the other, it seems uncontentious that knowingly being infectious places on one moral duties and obligations. How can we proceed? The obvious way forward is to see our duty not to infect others as more or less strong because it is overridable. In other words, the strength of our duties and obligations around infecting others varies between cases, because they can be overridden by countervailing considerations. Some of the relevant considerations are fairly straightforward. Whether one is knowingly or unwittingly infectious matters. Our duties and obligations are greater the more serious is the disease (one ought to be more careful of passing on HIV than a cold). The virulence of the disease is important, too. Professional considerations that counteract the moral duty not to spread contagion are also relevant. For example, it is more justifiable for a firefighter to go work with a cold than for an academic or a nurse on an elderly ward. Whether the disease is so prevalent that others might well catch it, whatever one does, is important. The intention behind the spread of infection – whether, for example, it is done maliciously – is especially noteworthy.

So, the way to do justice to the duty and obligations in this area, whilst avoiding the over-demandingness problem, is to agree that there are considerations that ameliorate our risking infecting others. In fact, this is probably what commentators such as Harris and Holm had in mind all along, because there are various caveats in their apparently extreme position. One is their use of the phrase, *prima facie* duty – i.e., duties that we have on the face of it, or at first blush – which implies that any obligations here are overridable by other considerations. Also, the position they defend is that 'communicating a disease is to inflict a harm proportionate to the severity of the disease and its consequences'. Since this severity can vary, so can the amount of harm and, in turn, the moral seriousness of the disease transmission. Again, this implies that the moral seriousness of our obligations and derelictions of duty can vary between cases of infecting others.

The strong general duty and the decision to get vaccinated

Where does this leave the specific obligation to get vaccinated, as grounded in a duty not to infect others? The same moral pattern emerges here. There are some very strong duties and obligations. Suppose, for example, there is a very safe and effective vaccine, refusal of which is highly likely to result in risk of, or actual, transmission of a serious disease to others. In such a case the duty not to infect others is not overridden. So, this duty entails a moral obligation to participate in this mass immunization campaign. Not to get vaccinated would be unethical. But imagine a different case. Here, it is useful to recall the nature of the dissent from immunization programmes discussed earlier in this chapter, where the point was made that people can and do dissent on perfectly reasonable and principled grounds. One might dissent because the vaccine is known, or sincerely believed, to be dangerous. Others might dissent on ideological grounds; for example, a serious and reflective libertarian might dissent as an act of principled resistance to an immunization programme based on what they argue is an unjustifiable relationship between the State and its citizenry. In such cases, though the duty not to infect others does not go away, the ensuing obligations are compromised by relevant countervailing considerations (the dangers of vaccination, the sincere political commitments). It seems perfectly plausible in such cases that the duty does not give rise to a strong obligation to participate.

Consider an illustration to clarify the point. Suppose I agree that I have a duty not to infect others. Let's say that this translates into specific moral obligations, such as to stay off work because I have measles. Is it nonetheless morally permissible for me to dissent from the measles, mumps and rubella (MMR) programme by refusing to allow my child to be vaccinated? In some circumstances, the answer is, yes. Suppose, for example, that my decision comes just after the publication of research suggesting that this combination of vaccines puts children at risk of autism. I sincerely believe it not to be in my child's best interests to receive the vaccine. Most people would agree that this provides justification for my dissension. So, we can drive a wedge in between the duty not to infect others, on the one hand, and the obligation to participate in a mass immunization programme, on the other. The upshot is that there is no strict or straightforward entailment from one's duty not to infect others to one's moral obligation to be vaccinated.

Free-riding

The discussions in the preceding two sections are generally sceptical about coercive State immunization policies; yet there is still a hankering sense that one ought to participate in vaccination programmes and that not to do so is morally dubious. The approach taken in this section connects directly with this intuition by raising the issue of free-riding. Technically speaking, free-riders are defined as '[u]sually unintended beneficiaries of a socially provided public good for which they have made no contribution' (Haldane 2005: 316). So, free-riding is about enjoying shared benefits without making a contribution to, nor running the risks of, the production of those benefits. A simple example is taking a bus ride without paying: the free-rider gets the benefits of the bus service without contributing to its upkeep. The idea applies neatly to immunization, where the 'socially provided public good' is herd immunity from a vaccine-preventable disease: 'one might argue that the unimmunized are "free-riders" in the sense that they take the benefit of high immunization rates without exposing themselves to the risks unavoidably attendant upon attaining those rates' (Dare 1998: 145).

As in previous sections, a simple argument suggests itself: not to get immunized is to free-ride; free-riding is morally wrong; therefore, not to get immunized is morally wrong. Let's call this the free-riding argument. Before evaluating it, note that this argument has strong intuitive support because, as just mentioned, it is natural to feel that free-riding is selfish and calculating. On the other hand, it is not quite clear what would follow from endorsing the argument. The obvious thought is that, if immunization free-riding is morally wrong, it is permissible to coerce free-riders to participate in vaccination programmes. So, the argument counts in favour of compulsory vaccination. Note, though, that this would leave open the question as to which of the various ways to compel free-riders to participate in mass immunization programmes is best, with options ranging from the more heavy-handed, such as straightforward legislation, to the less Draconian, such as ensuring that people are forced to consider and declare their vaccination status.

Evaluating the free-riding argument

The rest of this section evaluates the free-riding argument, but note that the evaluation is selective, in two ways. First, of the numerous ways of discussing the argument, the one chosen here is to apply moral theories. Second, three of the moral theories that were discussed in Chapters 1 and 2 are applied, namely, consequentialism, deontology and virtue ethics. Others are relevant to the topic – for example, Verweij and Dawson (2004) have adapted principlism (see Chapter 2) to the ethics of immunization – nonetheless, each of the three theories chosen for consideration here has been applied to the ethics of immunization in the relevant literature, and the way they interact with one another is instructive. Specifically, a problem emerges from the application of these theories to the free-riding argument. The problem is two-fold. First, the way each of these three moral theories applies to the decision to immunize is contestable. Second, even if we could reach a consensus on how each of these theories applies, it is unlikely that they would pull in the same direction with regard to the ethics of immunization. The upshot is that the free-riding argument is, at best, inconclusive.

To work into this, consider an interesting discussion of the immunization free-rider problem in an important paper that raises a number of philosophical issues about mass immunization, and concludes:

On balance it seems to me that we can properly describe at least some non-immunizers as free-riders, but that their conduct is not morally objectionable. Given what seem to be plausible assumptions about attainable coverage rates, immunization programmes are able to tolerate a small rump of voluntary non-immunizers. (Dare 1998: 147)

Why does Dare think that voluntary non-immunization is free-riding, yet morally unobjectionable? He begins by considering the ethics of free-riding in general. He then claims that 'although the term free-riding may seem pejorative, not all free-riding is morally objectionable' (p. 145); also, he lists various non-decisive factors that influence the moral value of a case of free-riding, prominent in which is 'the extent to which non-participation threatens the project as a whole' (p. 146). When he focuses on immunization free-riding in particular, he suggests that,

given that free-riders in the immunization case do not significantly increase the costs of the scheme for others, significantly alter what contributors should do given their preference to immunize, and since the conduct of free-riders does not seem to threaten the attainment of the good of immunization, I see little ground to justify moral criticism of non-immunizers on the ground that they are free-riders. (P. 147)

Although he does not state so explicitly, Dare clearly takes a consequentialist approach to the issue. He assumes that the moral value of immunization free-riding – whether it is objectionable, whether moral criticism of immunization free-riders is justified, and so on – is determined by expected consequences concerning such things as the costs of the programme, the behaviour of contributors, and the attainment of herd immunity.

Dare's position is perfectly defensible. If the moral value of free-riding depends on the consequences of free-riding – and since various factors can affect the consequences of free-riding – free-riding is neither always nor necessarily morally objectionable. It will depend on the consequences. And immunization free-riding in particular is not so bad because, typically and predictably, vaccination programmes are not undermined by some degree of voluntary dissension. In fact, not only can consequentialism allow free-riding, it can positively require it. For example, if herd immunity to a vaccine-controllable disease is achieved by vaccinating 90 per cent of the population, it would be reprehensible to expose any more than 90 per cent to the risks of the vaccine. On utilitarian grounds, we ought to allow 10 per cent of the population to free-ride.

Two problems with Dare's view: consequentialism and deontology

In evaluating Dare's position it is worth making the rather obvious point that his utilitarian approach to mass immunization cuts both ways, depending on circumstances. In other words, whilst Dare uses utilitarianism to justify immunization free-riding, it can also be used to justify heavy coercion to participate in vaccination programmes involving dangerous vaccines, at least in certain circumstances:

> a rough-and-ready utilitarian calculation is probably what the authorities have in mind when they decide to use preventive measures regardless of the risk they are imposing on a certain number of people. If the public health officials of New York [faced with the 1947 smallpox outbreak] had decided *not* to vaccinate the inhabitants of the city, thousands of people would have lost their lives. As the immunization programme itself only caused four deaths, the greater evil would obviously have been its absence. (Häyry and Häyry 1989: 44)

There are two more important problems with Dare's view. The first stays within the consequentialist perspective on which it is based. The consequentialist's moral endorsement of immunization free-riding seems to rely on a rather basic act-utilitarian version of consequentialism. Here, we need to recall the consequentialist constraints on the pursuit of maximal health gain discussed in Chapter 1, where the point was made that there are more plausible and sophisticated versions of consequentialism than the simple act-utilitarian dictum, act so as to maximize utility. Act-utilitarians can take into account long-term and indirect consequences; also, there are versions of utilitarianism more sophisticated than act-utilitarianism, notably rule-utilitarianism. Arguably, on at least some such accounts, immunization free-riding is ruled out. To illustrate, it is plausible that the rule-utilitarian would denounce free-riding in general, and immunization free-riding in particular, because a rule such as 'make contributions, and take associated risks, commensurable with one's enjoyment of a public good' is one that would be sanctioned and enforced by society because to do so would maximize utility.

The second problem with Dare's position is that, whatever a consequentialist would or should say about immunization free-riding, there are strong non-consequentialist critiques of this type of action. Some of these point to a conclusion at odds with Dare's. The best example recalls the discussion of deontology in Chapter 2. Deontology is the non-consequentialist view that some kinds of actions are ruled out as immoral by their very nature. A case in point is the kind of action that is based on non-universalizable maxims, the first formulation of Kant's categorical imperative being, 'act only on that maxim which you can at the same time will to be a universal law'. As mentioned in Chapter 2, the obvious application of this dictum in public health ethics is to rule out free-riding. This is because free-riding is a matter of some people taking advantage of the contribution and risk taking of others. So, it is not possible for everyone to free-ride because, if they did, no one would be making the contributions and taking the risks necessary for creating the public or social good in question. Free-riding is, by definition, non-universalizable in the Kantian sense explained in Chapter 2. In turn, according to Kant's dictum, immunization free-riding is an action that is always morally wrong, by its very nature, and irrespective of consequences.

Clearly, this Kantian analysis of free-riding is directly at odds with Dare's view. And it is a very plausible analysis because it chimes well with the general moral intuition mentioned earlier that there is something fundamentally morally wrong with free-riding whatever its consequences: 'Despite the fact that refusers in such a situation do not harm either their own child or others, non-compliance will strike many as morally problematic' (Menzel 1995: 114). But, in turn, this deontological argument is problematic because how Kant's categorical imperative applies to immunization free-riding is contestable. Menzel (1995: 114) puts the point very nicely:

> The dissenters' argument seems not to pass the 'what if everyone did that?' test commonly used in such contexts of interactive cooperation.
>
> But as students of this general moral test and its complexities know full well, however, the matter is not quite so simple. First, what is the 'that' in the [query] 'what if everyone did that?'

In other words, the relevant moral test is universalizability (the 'what if everyone did that?' test), the idea being that dissenting from mass immunization programmes is immoral because it fails this test; however, whether it does fail the test depends on how *it* is described.

To explain how different descriptions of the act in question affect whether it is universalizable, consider a mistake that Menzel (1995: 114) seems to make (cf. Menzel 2002). He suggests that we can describe the action of refusing a vaccination in different ways, and on some descriptions, 'the "what if everyone did that?" challenge [to voluntary non-immunizers] is deflected'. But this is about re-describing the action in universalizable ways. In fact, the first formulation of the categorical imperative ('act only on that maxim which you can at the same time will to be a universal law') is about the universalizability of maxims, not actions (it rules out acting in ways that express non-universalizable maxims). So, the important point is not that the act of refusing a vaccination can be re-described; rather, that same action can plausibly be said to express different maxims, some of which are universalizable, others of which are not.

To illustrate, suppose one claims that the maxim that the action of dissenting expresses is, 'avoid risks that can be avoided because others take them'. This maxim obviously fails the universalizability test: how could everybody avoid risks that can be avoided because others take them? In turn, the action – i.e., dissenting – is morally wrong. But suppose parents refuse to allow their child to be immunized because they sincerely believe that the vaccine is an unnecessary danger. The maxim their dissenting action expresses is, 'do your utmost to protect your own children'. Is this maxim universalizable? Recalling terminology explained in Chapter 2, to universalize this maxim would commit one neither to a contradiction in conception nor to a contradiction in the will. Since the maxim is universalizable, the action is not proscribed. Of course, there is room here for sophistry and trickery because one might say that a dubious action expresses a universalizable maxim in order to avoid a Kantian proscription. But dissenting from vaccination programmes does not seem to be like this because many dissenters could accurately describe their actions in terms of a maxim such as, 'protect your children'.

Virtue ethics

So far, then, the problems with the free-riding argument are mounting up. Applications of consequentialism and deontology are problematic, and certainly do not point clearly in a single moral direction. Now we can add a further complication by looking at the argument from the perspective supplied by our third moral theory, namely, virtue ethics. There is a clear reference to this in Dare's article:

> Concern with whether or not non-immunizers go out of their way to take advantage of immunization programmes leads us into worries about the character of non-immunizers. Plainly this can be relevant to moral assessment. (P. 146)

Another simple argument suggests itself: to immunization free-ride is to lack virtue; we should act in accordance with the virtues; therefore, immunization free-riding is wrong. Let's call this the virtue argument.

But, yet again, this is both more complicated than it first appears and, ultimately, inconclusive. Anyone who voluntarily refuses to participate in a successful mass immunization programme is free-riding, as that class of actions is technically defined, because they all enjoy the benefits of a public good (herd immunity) without making the contribution (getting vaccinated) or taking necessary risks (i.e., those associated with the vaccine). But whether their dissension reveals a vicious character – and, in turn, how convincing the virtue ethics argument against immunization free-riding is – depends on the motivation or intention behind refusing vaccination. Here, we need some more details about dissension. Consider three categories of cases of vaccine refusal (in reality the situation is no doubt more complex, but these illustrate the salient points). First, there are those who refuse a vaccination with the express intention of getting the benefits of herd immunity without any contribution or risk taking. Second, there are those who refuse vaccinations on unprincipled grounds, such as ignorance and apathy. Third, there are those who dissent on principled grounds, including religious and philosophical convictions.

Taking these in turn, what about the dissenter who refuses a vaccine with the express intention of free-riding? There is a red herring here that trades on the distinction between the morality of an act and the blameworthiness of the agent, i.e., between whether an action is right or wrong, on the one hand, and how good or bad the agent is who committed the act, on the other. Given this distinction, one might suggest that the virtue argument is really about the blameworthiness of the agent, as opposed to the moral value of the act. Our first type of dissenter, i.e., someone who expressly free-rides on a successful mass immunization programme, is morally blameworthy. But, arguably, the action is not morally wrong: recall, for example, Dare's position, on which immunization free-riding is morally unobjectionable up to a point (the point at which it has bad consequences). So, one might say, this kind of self-conscious, calculated immunization free-riding is permissible on act-utilitarian grounds, but the agent is blameworthy because they lack virtue.

This is a red herring because it begs the question against virtue ethics. In other words, a large part of the point of virtue ethics is to close the gap between the moral assessment of agents, on the one hand, and of their actions on the other. The thought behind virtue ethics is that the praiseworthiness and blameworthiness of the agent establishes or determines the rightness and wrongness of their actions. So, to pull the two – i.e., actions and agents – apart in this way is quite counter to the theory being applied, namely, virtue ethics. Referring again to the first category of deliberate free-riders, suppose there is a relatively safe, effective and convenient vaccine that someone refuses simply because they self-consciously and deliberately work out they can free-ride. Since this is selfish, it is wrong; i.e., the blameworthiness of the agent establishes the wrongness of the action. In turn, the government is, arguably, within its rights to enforce participation.

What about the second kind of dissenter, who refuses a vaccine on unprincipled grounds, such as apathy? This is complicated by the fact that, unlike the previous case, they do not set out to free-ride. As Dare put it, they do not 'go out of their way to take advantage of immuniza-tion programmes'. Nonetheless, as Dare (1998: 146) points out, one might well consider the traits in question, such as apathy, that underlie the refusal to vaccinate, to be vicious. So, even though the dissension is not directly linked to a vice such as selfishness, it is grounded in a character flaw. Again, as such it is morally dubious, and, in turn, one might argue that the State is within its rights to compel people to face up to this and participate.

So far, then, there is cogent support for the virtue argument. The problem concerns the third kind of dissenter, who refuses a vaccine on principled grounds. We have already encountered various such grounds. For some people, participation in a mass immunization pro-gramme is counter to their deeply held religious convictions. Others find that it contradicts their secular views about science, philosophy or politics. For example, some dissenters question the scientific meth-odologies that provide the data on which vaccine programmes are based; some question the understanding of concepts such as health, harm and benefit at work in mass immunization campaigns; some reject a campaign on the grounds that it requires and bolsters an unjustifiable relationship between the State and its citizenry. Of course, one might castigate such people for their odd and unconvincing views. But the point at issue here is not that the principles on which people dissent are questionable; rather, it is whether the refusal of a vaccina-tion on principled grounds supports the virtue argument.

The obvious point to make here is that, far from expressing a vicious character, principled dissension from mass immunization programmes might be taken to express virtue. For example, dissension can require loyalty to, and steadfastness in the face of pressure to go against, one's deeply held convictions. Of course, this is not always convincing: a dissenter who claims to be acting on a conviction that they have not really thought through lacks some intellectual virtues, for example.

Nonetheless, it is plausible that the refusing of a vaccine can not only not lack, but actually express, virtue. Now suppose that we endorse a blanket policy of compulsory immunization, based on the virtue argument against the first two kinds of free-riders just discussed. This would be unjust because it would also impact on this third kind of free-rider, the principled dissenter. In other words, however much support for compulsory immunization is provided by the unprincipled dissenters' lack of virtue, the policy is dubious because of its impact on the principled dissenters.

Although there is not space to explore this interesting area more fully, at least one further line of argument can be indicated. Perhaps this problem with the virtue argument can be met by a policy of exemptions to vaccination on grounds of conscientious objection. In other words, we aim to rule out free-riding grounded directly by vices such as selfishness, and indirectly by vices such as apathy, whilst allowing principled dissension on philosophical and religious grounds. Suffice to say that vaccination exemption policies are fraught with theoretical and practical difficulties. May and Silverman (2005) have provided a clear and stimulating discussion of theoretical issues, centring on the dilemma between retaining herd immunity and allowing an exemption option. Salmon et al. (1999) take a more practical approach, providing an empirical analysis of the health consequences of vaccination exemption. No doubt some of these theoretical and practical concerns about an exemption option can be met. Nonetheless, they indicate the general problem with the virtue argument: it is simply not the case that all refusers of vaccines lack virtue, because the reality of mass immunization programmes leaves plenty of room for virtuous dissent.

That voluntary dissension from mass immunization programmes is wrong because it is free-riding is a powerful idea that would support coercive policies in this area of public health. But the idea is vexed. The problem is multi-layered. The application of moral theory to the issue is both unclear and clearly conflicting. Different applications of the same theory, and applications of different theories, pull in various directions. So, it does not seem feasible to ground immunization policy on the free-riding argument.

Concluding remarks

This chapter has discussed vaccination ethics. The central dilemma is whether to make participation in mass immunization programmes voluntary or mandatory. Two perspectives on this dilemma – that of the State and that of the individual – were distinguished. Then, three lines of enquiry were pursued. Is compulsory participation justified by appeal to the harm principle, a strong general duty not to infect others, and the proscription against free-riding? Although there is much to be said for each of these, in the end none provides a very strong argument for mandatory participation in mass immunization programmes. The roots of the problem with coercion lie quite deep, in the natures of mass immunization and dissension: mass immunization programmes are very complex affairs that invite sincere, thoughtful and principled dissension. Forcing people to get vaccinated is not like forcing people to drive on the right side of the road, because the risks and benefits of vaccination are contestable, the phenomenology of vaccination is complex, and features such as parental rights are influential. Hence, the drift of the arguments in this chapter is towards scepticism about the State coercing people to get vaccinated.

10   Screening

Immunization, as discussed in the previous chapter, is a major form of primary prevention. By contrast, secondary prevention aims to 'identify and treat asymptomatic persons who have already developed risk factors or preclinical disease but in whom the condition is not clinically apparent' (US Preventive Services Task Force 1996: xli). Screening is an important form of secondary prevention that has developed into a major branch of public health; the ethics of screening is the focus of this chapter, which is in three parts. First, screening is explained and described. Then, generic issues – ethical considerations that apply to any screening programme – are discussed. The third and final section of the chapter is an in-depth analysis of one very important facet of screening, namely, benefit.

Screening programmes

The basic idea behind screening is very simple: identify people who will benefit from early detection of risk factors for, or the onset of, a disease. But this simplicity is deceptive because there is now a very diverse range of current and feasible screening programmes that differ in terms of who to screen, how to screen, and what to screen for. This proliferation is largely due to the fact that screening has proved extremely beneficial, but it is also due to developments in related fields, notably genetic medicine, that encourage screening programmes different from the standard model of early detection of a clinical disease for the sake of more effective medical treatment. As a result, screening has become a very complicated matter, ethically speaking, as different – but equally deep and troubling – questions arise concerning the justifiability of diverse screening programmes.

Before describing the current field of screening, it is worth clarifying the relationship between health screening and testing. The distinction is usually drawn along the following lines: screening comprises programmes aimed at a population, no member of which is thought to be at greater risk than any other of the screened-for condition; by contrast, testing comprises a procedure performed on an individual, usually in a doctor–patient relationship, who has been identified as being at high risk of the tested-for condition. Secondly, testing confirms a condition, whereas, often, screening only indicates a heightened risk of it, confirmation requiring a further diagnostic test. As a consequence of such considerations, '[m]uch has been made of the distinction between *screening* and *testing*' (Fost 1992: 2813), not least in ethical debates which tend to be categorized as centring on public health ethics questions about screening versus medical and bioethical questions about testing.

But, as Fost rightly goes on to explain, the distinction between the two is more vague and less clear-cut than this. They merge in certain cases, notably those involving pre-implantation genetic diagnosis (PGD) in which embryos are checked *in vitro* for a faulty gene before being implanted in the womb. PGD has the hallmarks of testing: specific embryos are selected because one or both of the parents are carriers, and the test is diagnostic (it confirms the presence of the faulty gene). Nonetheless, this is often called 'embryo screening'. A classic case is embryo screening for inherited bowel cancer, which involves PGD to detect familial adenomatous polyposis (FAP). Also, screening and testing have the same basic aim, namely, to produce beneficial health information. All screening programmes involve testing because members of a screened population are tested for the condition in question. And a common response to a positive screening result is a further test. Some tests can now be considered as screening programmes because they have become widespread and standard practice.

Points such as these lead Fost to conclude: 'I do not find this distinction a particularly useful one in considering the ethical issues' (1992: 2813; see, also, Nuffield Council on Bioethics 1993: 3). It is worth bearing this in mind. Nonetheless, there is a simple basic structure common to, and distinctive of, paradigmatic cases of health screening programmes. It has four components. First, the screened population. The point to stress here is that screening is of an asymptomatic population. In other words, a screening programme is aimed at detecting people who have a predisposition to a condition, or who already have the screened-for condition but in an early, preclinical stage, as opposed to people in whom the condition has given rise to symptoms. Second, the condition. Some screened-for conditions – Down's syndrome, hearing impairment in children, breast and cervical cancer, etc. – are well known; but, as we shall see, much of the current debate about the ethics of screening centres on whether to introduce screening for new, more contentious conditions such as late-onset genetic disorders and mental illnesses. Third, the screening test. All screening programmes require a way of investigating the screened population for the condition in question. These can be more or less intrusive and onerous for the screenees, so a traditional concern about programmes is whether the harms caused by a screening test outweigh benefits to screenees. Finally, the treatment. Some screening programmes identify individuals as needing treatment; others identify at-risk individuals who require a further diagnostic test prior to treatment to establish whether they have the condition in question.

Numerous and very diverse actual and feasible health screening programmes have developed from this simple structure. It is important to attempt some form of classification of these in order to make sense of this complex field. Here, two classificatory dimensions are described. First, health screening programmes can be classified in terms of the chronology of a human life-cycle. Second, health screening can be divided into non-genetic and genetic programmes. These are only two ways of describing health screening, and they do not map neatly on to one another; nonetheless, they help to manage the material, and both are especially useful in identifying the main ethical aspects of health screening.

Life-cycle

In surveying health screening chronologically – i.e., in terms of the typical life-cycle of human beings – four categories are especially important: foetuses, neonates, children, and adults. One might say that there is a fifth, namely, embryo screening, but as we saw a moment ago, this is a good example of how blurred the distinction between screening and testing is: embryo 'screening' can be thought of as pre-implantation genetic diagnosis (PGD), i.e., genetic testing, because only embryos at heightened risk of a genetic defect are tested, and the aim of the test is diagnostic.

Antenatal screening programmes are now very well established and aim at detecting conditions in both the mother and the unborn baby. To take each in turn, screening for maternal disease involves monitoring pregnancies with the aim of identifying conditions in asymptomatic women that threaten the health of their unborn baby. Such conditions include anaemia, HIV infection, diabetes, urinary tract infection, syphilis and high blood pressure. Having detected the condition, treatment is implemented in order to reduce the effect of the disease on the foetus. Also, the mother's immunity to rubella is checked, so that any non-immune mothers can be vaccinated after delivery; and the baby of a mother found to have hepatitis B can be immunized soon after birth to prevent their becoming infected.

Antenatal screening of unborn babies for foetal abnormality is now a very routine aspect of maternity care. There are two main groups of programmes. The first uses ultrasound examination to reveal structural abnormalities of the unborn baby – notably, abnormalities of the heart, spine, face and brain – as well as neural tube defects. In this case, early detection allows couples to make an informed choice about continuing the pregnancy; in some cases, treatment of the baby can be planned for soon after delivery. Second, antenatal screening is done by a blood test on the mother to detect blood disorders in the unborn baby, such as sickle cell disorder, thalassaemia, or haemolytic disease. Both methods – blood tests and ultrasound scans – may indicate a high risk of a baby being affected by Down's syndrome. In this case, a further diagnostic test (chorionic villus sampling or amniocentesis) can be undertaken, depending on how far the pregnancy has progressed, to confirm the presence or absence of the condition. (For an interesting and insightful reconstruction – informed by social constructivism and feminism – of the various ways in which antenatal genetic testing and screening can be understood, see Lippman 1991; see, also, Parker 1995.)

Neonatal screening programmes are designed to detect disabling congenital disorders in newborn babies as soon as possible after birth in order to ameliorate the impact on the child's quality of life. Two well-established programmes can serve to illustrate neonatal screening. First, a blood spot is taken from the baby's heel about 6–7 days after birth, and tested for phenylketonuria (PKU) and congenital hypothyroidism. Other conditions that can be tested for by blood spot include cystic fibrosis and sickle cell disorder. Second, babies have a routine general physical examination after birth to ensure that there are no visible malformations. Specifically, eye conditions (such as cataracts) and heart defects are screened for; hips are checked for developmental dysphasia, and testes for cryptorchidism.

Childhood screening, i.e., after the neonatal period, is also a well-established aspect of mother and child health (Elliman et al. 2002). All babies have a routine general physical examination at eight weeks which takes the same form as that in the neonatal period. Other targets of childhood screening programmes include hearing impairment and vision defects. Both are the subject of extensive literatures. For example, the effectiveness of a school-entry hearing screen has been researched (Henderson and Newton 2000; cf. Davis et al. 1997), as have current and proposed screening programmes for ophthalmic disorders and visual deficits (Rahi et al. 2001). It has been argued that childhood screening generates distinctive ethical worries: 'The most important ethical problem with [childhood screening programmes] is that the process of identifying the benefits and harms is complicated and incomplete, but this information is not communicated to parents' (Stewart-Brown 1999: 119). Also, the rather haphazard development and provision of childhood screening cause concern, and critique of both audio and visual childhood screening programmes focuses on the evidence base for their effectiveness. A particularly contentious aspect of childhood screening is whether to implement programmes for early detection of developmental and behavioural disorders, including speech and language delay, autism, and disruptive behaviour disorders such as attention-deficit/hyperactivity disorders (ADHD).

Finally, various categories of screening programmes aimed at adults can be usefully distinguished. First, there are the relatively straightforward cases of early detection of a condition in an asymptomatic population. Paradigmatic cases include the well-known screening programmes for breast and cervical cancers. There are numerous proposed screening programmes, some of which are under investigation, others of which are at the pilot stage. Some particularly contentious proposals involve whom to screen (for example, would-be immigrants for communicable diseases; Coker 2004) and what to screen for (whether primary care practitioners should screen women for domestic abuse, for example; Ramsay et al. 2002). But genetic screening programmes of adults – such as those that aim at couples starting a family, and those that aim at ascertaining genetic carrier status in the general population – are the most interesting and contentious. This brings us on to genetic screening.

Genetic screening

General advances in genetic medicine, and more specific achievements such as the human genome project, have increased our understanding of the genetic basis of diseases (Epstein 2000; Vogel and Motulsky 2002). In turn, this has created new medical opportunities, including screening populations for a disease-related genetic component (Khoury et al. 2000, 2003). It is important to clarify what distinguishes a genetic from a non-genetic screening programme. In a somewhat dated, but still very useful, report, the Nuffield Council on Bioethics (1993: 3) defined genetic screening as 'a search in a population to identify individuals who may have, or be susceptible to, a serious genetic disease, or who, though not at risk themselves, as gene carriers may be at risk of having children with that genetic disease'.

Genetic disorders are of three kinds: single gene (or monogenic) disorders, multifactorial (or polygenic) disorders, and chromosomal disorders. Single gene disorders are caused by inheriting an altered gene. Well-known examples include cystic fibrosis, PKU, Duchenne muscular dystrophy and haemophilia. Multifactorial genetic disorders are more complex in two respects: they result from mutations in multiple genes, as opposed to the inheritance of a single altered gene; and such mutations combine with environmental factors to produce the condition. Consequently, multifactorial genetic disorders have a much more complicated basis than do single gene disorders. In turn, this makes them more difficult to study, screen for, and treat. Examples of multifactorial genetic disorders include coronary heart disease, diabetes and some cancers. Chromosomal disorders are caused in two ways: an entire chromosome is added or missing (for example, Down's syndrome), or chromosomal material is rearranged (how serious the clinical effects of this are depends on whether there has been a net loss or gain of chromosomal material, as opposed to an exchange between or within chromosomes).

There are three main categories of genetic screenees: people who have a genetic disease, people who have a predisposition to adult-onset or late-onset genetic disorders, and people who are unaffected carriers of a genetic defect. Different ethical issues are raised by each of these. The first might seem least problematic. For example, as mentioned, in countries such as the UK, neonates are currently screened by blood spot for PKU so the condition can be identified early enough to ameliorate its effects on the child. But there are more contentious versions of such programmes, such as those in which the screened population comprises foetuses at risk of being aborted (this is discussed at length in the last section of this chapter). Adult-onset or late-onset disorders are those diseases that tend to manifest themselves after childhood and adolescence, in later life. Examples include the major current causes of death and disability in the West, notably heart disease, stroke, cancer and diabetes – all of which tend to arise during or after middle-age – plus neurogenetic disorders such as Huntington's disease, Alzheimer's and some forms of ataxia, which tend to manifest themselves in the elderly. Finally, population screening programmes for Tay–Sachs disease and cystic fibrosis are examples of genetic screening to detect carrier status amongst people unaffected by the condition. As we shall discuss in the last section of this chapter, such programmes raise distinctive ethical questions concerning the purpose of screening since, arguably, one objective of such programmes is to acquire genetic information *per se*, as opposed to the traditional rationale of providing the patient with earlier, so more effective, treatment.

Apart from whom to screen, genetic medicine has motivated a lively debate about what to screen for. A central point here is that it appears likely that some mental illnesses, notably psychotic disorders such as schizophrenia, are partly genes-based. If so, ought we to implement genetic screening programmes aimed at early detection of individuals at risk of developing the condition? It is worth noting how vexed the question is: on the one hand, schizophrenia is a condition that is bad for the patient and others, and for which there are effective interventions; on the other, and as discussed in Chapter 6, there are well-established worries about the status of mental illnesses, and whether such a screening programme relies on overbearing techniques of health surveillance and social control. Screening for a predisposition to anti-social behaviour traits is even more vexed. Criminality, for example, clearly causes serious harm; if we could, should we screen for early genetic detection of a criminal predisposition, or is this an intolerable burden on the erstwhile innocent (Rosen 2000)?

Finally, it should be noted that much of the ethical debate about genetic screening is hypothetical in that many of the programmes under discussion are only feasible in principle; we neither do, nor could, implement them because of the inchoate state of genetic medicine (Godard et al. 2003). However, this does not nullify the debate. Striking successes in genetics make it very likely that such screening programmes will become a reality, and, as we shall see, they present such new and difficult ethical challenges that it is important to discuss them even at this stage in the development of genetic medicine. The list of main ethical issues generated by genetic screening is well established and frequently cited. Bailey et al. (2005: 1890) sum it up neatly:

'concerns about privacy of information, insurance discrimination, stigmatization of individuals or groups, psychological distress, endangerment of the parent–child bond, lack of adequate follow-up to testing, and selective abortion'. Later in this chapter we focus in on some of the ethical issues in genetic screening; first, though, some issues generic to screening need to be discussed.

Generic issues

General harms

For all their diversity, all screening programmes are designed to offer the benefits of early detection, but bring with them some risk of harm (Juth and Munthe 2012; Delatycki 2012). One oft-cited set of harms incurred by health screening includes such things as the inconvenience of participating in a screening programme, the unpleasantness of the relevant test, and an anxious wait for results (Sox 1998). How important are such features? For one thing, harms of this kind are more important in some screening programmes than in others. For example, it would not be surprising if waiting for the results of a screening test for HIV or Down's syndrome proved more onerous than waiting for the results of a test for secondary diabetes, because of the nature of these conditions. Also, the screenee's personality and circumstances inform how great such harms are: screening involving a blood test is more harmful to a needle-phobic than it is to me, and more inconvenient to someone living in a remote rural area than to someone living in a town and near a clinic.

One thought about such harms that naturally occurs is that most medical interventions other than screening, such as medical testing and clinical treatments, are also inconvenient, unpleasant and anxiety provoking, but are, nonetheless, generally seen as perfectly well justified by their beneficial outcomes. Here, the distinctive nature of secondary prevention needs to be borne in mind. Screening is of an asymptomatic population. Typically, the vast majority of people screened turn out not to have the condition in question. In their cases, harms such as inconvenience, unpleasantness and anxiety are offset only by reassurance that they are free of the screened-for condition. But, usually, most of the screenees had not considered that they might have the relevant condition prior to being investigated, so the reassurance is not experienced as a great benefit. By contrast, similar harms incurred in medical testing and clinical treatment are offset by what is actually experienced as a massive benefit by a patient who knew they were, or were very likely to be, ill, and fully appreciate early diagnosis and treatment.

Sensitivity and specificity

The kinds of harms discussed so far are relatively mild. More worrying is the serious damage that can ensue from inaccurate screening results (McCormick 1996: 620; Elmore et al. 1998). This introduces a second issue generic to health screening: screening processes are always in a distinctive way less than perfect. Screening produces four kinds of results:

- True positive: person with the disease is identified as having it.
- False positive: person without the disease is identified as having it.
- True negative: person without the disease is identified as not having it.
- False negative: person with the disease is identified as not having it.

So, we can get the results of screening right in two ways: a person with the disease is found to have it; a person without the disease is found not to have it. But we can get them wrong in two ways, too: a person without the disease is told they have it; a person with the disease is told they do not have it. This is a distinctive feature of screening (even medical testing – the closest bedfellow of screening – tends to be more accurate than screening). In the light of this, screening programmes can be more or less 'sensitive' and 'specific':

- Sensitivity: the proportion of those people with the disease who are correctly identified as such;
- Specificity: the proportion of those people who do not have the disease who are correctly identified as such.

To clarify, imagine a screened population of ten, of which three members have the disease. A perfectly sensitive and specific screening programme tells the three people with the disease that they have it (sensitivity), and tells the other seven that they do not (specificity).

However, screening programmes are, typically, only more or less – as opposed to perfectly – sensitive and specific. This creates a dilemma. Making a programme more sensitive increases the likelihood of false positives because, by trying to make sure that everyone with the disease gets identified, people without the disease are more likely to be identified as having it. Making a programme more specific increases the likelihood of false negatives because, by trying to make sure that everyone without the disease gets identified, people with the disease are more likely to be identified as not having it. So, programmes are adjusted to trade off sensitivity and specificity.

One way of adjusting a screening programme is by altering the 'threshold'. A threshold is a cut-off point above which a screenee is positive and below which they are negative. Usually, the threshold is a simple numerical or statistical figure, for example, a blood cholesterol level of such-and-such, a body-mass index (BMI) of such-and-such, such-and-such a percentage likelihood of Down's syndrome. Roughly, we increase sensitivity by lowering the threshold, and increase specificity by increasing the threshold. Recalling the screened population of ten, of whom three have the disease, the central question is whether the priority is to identify the three with the disease, or to identify the seven without it. By lowering the threshold we increase sensitivity and thereby identify the three, but we might well tell some of the seven they have the condition when, on further testing, it turns out that they do not; i.e., there will be false positives. By increasing the threshold we increase specificity and thereby successfully identify the seven who do not have the condition, but we might well tell some of the three that they do not have the condition when in fact they do; i.e., there will be false negatives.

The threshold for a screening programme is obviously important because it triggers further investigation or treatment. And, as mentioned, the resultant trade-off between sensitivity and specificity is usually put in terms of a dilemma in discussions of screening. This gives the impression that there is a deep ethical problem here. Is there? On the one hand, it is true that, whilst ideally a threshold is set by sound epidemiology – i.e., our understanding of the risks associated with the disease in question should dictate the threshold – it can be influenced by much more dubious factors, including political requirements to be seen to be doing something about high profile conditions, changes in public and media perceptions of a disease, and the availability of resources to treat the screened-for condition (Shickle and Chadwick 1994). But it is worth emphasizing again that this problem depends on the programme in question. Some screening tests are more specific and sensitive than others. For example, screening for HIV would be highly specific and sensitive. By contrast, screening for diabetes and hypertension requires setting a variable threshold in order to distinguish positive and negative results.

Of course, thresholds have to be set, and we can get them wrong. But we should bear in mind that, whatever the public perception, medicine generally is a more or less inexact science. More importantly, perhaps what the sensitivity–specificity trade-off best illustrates is that the development of a screening programme is an iterative, as opposed to a 'once and for all', process. In other words, the way to get health screening programmes right is to repeatedly review and amend them in the light of such factors as new medical and epidemiological data, changes in resource availability and public attitudes, and so on. We ought to be prepared to review and revise details of a screening programme. This is nicely illustrated by, but not restricted to, the threshold issue: it also includes such aspects as how to consent, test and inform screenees (Grimes and Schultz 2002).

A further point in favour of this assessment of the dilemma between sensitivity and specificity is that it is often not so hard to discern grounds for prioritizing one or the other. For example, Shickle and Chadwick (1994: 13) suggest that high specificity is desirable when the screened-for condition is associated with anxiety or stigma, investigations are especially onerous (time consuming, painful, expensive), there are other means of sufficiently early detection, and treatment (especially if it produces notable harmful side effects) is offered without further investigation. By contrast, sensitivity is preferable when the adverse consequences of missed diagnosis are very bad for the individual (for example, early treatment is significantly more effective than later) or society (in the case of communicable diseases, for example), and the adverse consequences of a false positive are not so bad (for example, the period of anxiety is short because other investigations will confirm the diagnosis before treatment anyway). (For further details on screening, sensitivity, and threshold – and other, related notions such as the predictive value of a programme – see Jaeschke et al. 1994a, 1994b; Gostin 2000: 191; cf. Choi 1993.)

General criteria for ethical screening

An important issue generic to health screening is whether there are criteria that any health screening programme must meet in order to be ethically acceptable. Of the various important sets of criteria that have been proposed (Cochrane and Holland 1971; Cadman et al. 1984; Kizer 1991), two landmark publications are most notable. Wilson and Jungner (1968) proposed a framework for evaluating screening tests that includes the following:

- The screened-for disease should be an important health problem.
- The disease should have a recognizable latent or early symptomatic stage.
- The natural history of the disease, including development from latent to declared disease, should be adequately understood.
- There should be a suitable test or examination.

- The test should be acceptable to the population.
- There should be an accepted and effective treatment.
- The policy concerning whom to treat as patients should be agreed on.
- Facilities for diagnosis and treatment should be available.
- Case finding should be continuous, or ongoing, not 'once and for all'.
- The cost of case finding (including diagnosis and treatment of patients diagnosed) should be economically balanced in relation to possible expenditures on medical care as whole.

These principles have been frequently quoted, influential, heavily criticized, and reworked (Goel 2001). Most importantly, they became somewhat outdated because they were drawn up before the developments in genetic medicine that have given rise to the prospect of genetic screening. Consequently, more recent and appropriate ethical criteria for health screening programmes have been suggested, many of which are geared specifically to genetic screening (for a summary, see Godard et al. 2003: 51–3). One particularly cogent set worth citing is by the UK's National Screening Committee (National Screening Committee 1998). The NSC's First Report in 1998 published seventeen 'criteria for appraising the viability, effectiveness and appropriateness of a screening programme'; these were expanded in the Second Report of 2003, and updated in 2009:

The condition

1. The condition should be an important health problem.
2. The epidemiology and natural history of the condition, including development from latent to declared disease, should be adequately understood and there should be a detectable risk factor, disease marker, latent period or early symptomatic stage.
3. All the cost-effective primary prevention interventions should have been implemented as far as practicable.
4. If the carriers of a mutation are identified as a result of screening, the natural history of people with this status should be understood, including the psychological implications.

The test

5. There should be a simple, safe, precise and validated screening test.
6. The distribution of test values in the target population should be known and a suitable cut-off level defined and agreed.

7. The test should be acceptable to the population.
8. There should be an agreed policy on the further diagnostic investigation of individuals with a positive test result and on the choices available to those individuals.
9. If the test is for mutations, the criteria used to select the subset of mutations to be covered by screening, if all possible mutations are not being tested, should be clearly set out.

The treatment

10. There should be an effective treatment or intervention for patients identified through early detection, with evidence of early treatment leading to better outcomes than late treatment.
11. There should be agreed evidence-based policies covering which individuals should be offered treatment and the appropriate treatment to be offered.
12. Clinical management of the condition and patient outcomes should be optimized in all health care providers prior to participation in a screening programme.

The screening programme

13. There should be evidence from high quality Randomized Controlled Trials that the screening programme is effective in reducing mortality or morbidity. Where screening is aimed solely at providing information to allow the person being screened to make an 'informed choice' (e.g., Down's syndrome, cystic fibrosis carrier screening), there must be evidence from high quality trials that the test accurately measures risk. The information that is provided about the test and its outcome must be of value and readily understood by the individual being screened.
14. There should be evidence that the complete screening programme (test, diagnostic procedures, treatment/intervention) is clinically, socially and ethically acceptable to health professionals and the public.
15. The benefit from the screening programme should outweigh the physical and psychological harm (caused by the test, diagnostic procedures and treatment).
16. The opportunity cost of the screening programme (including testing, diagnosis and treatment, administration, training and quality assurance) should be economically balanced in relation to expenditure on medical care as a whole (i.e., value for money).

Assessment against this criteria should have regard to evidence from cost–benefit and/or cost-effectiveness analyses and have regard to the effective use of available resource.
17. All other options for managing the condition should have been considered (e.g., improving treatment, providing other services), to ensure that no more cost-effective intervention could be introduced or current interventions increased within the resources available.
18. There should be a plan for managing and monitoring the screening programme and an agreed set of quality assurance standards.
19. Adequate staffing and facilities for testing, diagnosis, treatment and programme management should be available prior to the commencement of the screening programme.
20. Evidence-based information, explaining the consequences of testing, investigation and treatment, should be made available to potential participants to assist them in making an informed choice.
21. Public pressure for widening the eligibility criteria for reducing the screening interval, and for increasing the sensitivity of the testing process, should be anticipated. Decisions about these parameters should be scientifically justifiable to the public.
22. If screening is for a mutation, the programme should be acceptable to people identified as carriers and to other family members.

Evaluating general ethical criteria

How convincing are such lists of ethical criteria for screening programmes? On the one hand, they are rather blunt instruments. Partly, the problem is that it would not be appropriate to require that all of, say, the NSC's criteria are fully met by all health screening programmes. To do so would be quite unrealistic, for at least three reasons. First, the criteria are too stringent, if taken literally (*all* the cost-effective primary prevention interventions (3); *all* other options (17)?). Most of the criteria include vague, contestable terms, such as 'important' (1), 'acceptable' (7), and 'adequate' (19). And some contain demands that are question-begging; for example, the list implies that epidemiology (2) and health economics (16) are sciences for which there is a settled consensus on the best techniques and research methodologies, when, in fact, they are more inchoate and contested than this.

Nonetheless, such lists serve a number of more general purposes. Published and frequently cited ethical criteria play a role similar to professional guidelines and codes of conduct familiar from other contexts: they help focus individuals and organizations on the ethical dimension of screening, including publicizing principal ethical challenges and requirements. Revisiting and revising ethical criteria can result in the coalescence of opinion on the main problems and principles of ethical health screening. Such criteria provide a context in which to consider and debate good screening practice. And published criteria can be useful in the training of future professionals (it is easy to see how the NSC's list could form part of relevant public health curricula, for example). Already, a lot of good work has been done in assessing programmes against published criteria (Rouse and Adab 2001).

A charitable view of ethical criteria is that, like professional guidelines and codes of conduct, they are to be applauded for their general contribution to the ethics of health screening, as opposed to being taken too literally. However, one final comment worth making recalls the moral theory discussed in Part I. The point was made in Chapter 1 that utilitarianism is the moral theory that drives public health in general. Public health is a utilitarian endeavour because it aims to produce utility in the form of health gain. The NSC's ethical criteria for screening are basically utilitarian in that they are either explicitly or implicitly driven by the assumption that the ethical soundness of a screening programme is determined by its consequences. Even criteria such as numbers 7 and 14 can be interpreted along utilitarian lines as grounded in the view that the effectiveness of screening programmes is enhanced by their acquiring a public mandate.

As clarified in Chapter 1, utilitarianism is a noteworthy moral theory that captures an important ethical dimension. So, the utilitarian basis of the NSC's criteria is not dubious or inappropriate *per se*. Nonetheless, the strategy of Part I was to take 'simple and unqualified' utilitarianism in public health as our starting point, then reveal how this is offset by alternative theoretical considerations. For example, moral perspectives supplied by non-consequentialist theories such as deontology and principlism are different from, and sometimes at odds with, a utilitarian approach in public health. Arguably, such alternative perspectives are understated in the National Screening Committee's criteria which, as a result, come across as rather naïvely utilitarian.

Take, for example, an issue such as consent (O'Hagan 1991; Austoker 1999; British Medical Association 2005). A right to consent can be grounded in utilitarianism. But it is more natural to take consent to be a non-consequentialist, i.e., deontological, medical ethical principle: in other words, consent is grounded in the fact that the nature of the action of treating a competent individual against their will makes it morally wrong (Chaloner 2003). What of the screenee's right to consent to participate in a screening programme? It would be natural to think that there is no problem here because one consents to participation simply by participating; i.e., turning up to be investigated implies consent to be screened. But things are surely more complicated than this. The problem is not so much that we screen individuals incapable of consent – children, for example – because it is often considered ethical to test and treat incompetent patients for their own good; rather, the problem is that competent screenees tend to feel disempowered when it comes to refusing to be screened: 'Health professionals may respect the decisions of those who decline the offer of screening, not coercing them into compliance, but those who decide against participation will carry a label of societal deviance unless great efforts have been made to avoid this' (Clarke 1998: 401). For example, when a health visitor begins to screen a baby or a letter arrives 'inviting' a woman to attend for a screening investigation, consent is so obviously presumed that refusal seems impossible. Furthermore, the result of a screening investigation tends to get a juggernaut of diagnostic testing and/or treatment going in a way that feels out of the control of the patient.

How well do the NSC ethical criteria capture such deontological themes as consent to participate in a screening programme? On the one hand, one might assume that they are implicitly included in criteria such as number 14: a programme that flouts the right to consent would be unacceptable to the public. But public acceptability and respecting the right to consent are not the same thing. And it is easy to imagine a health screening programme that becomes broadly accepted despite involving some measure of coercion to participate. So, the worry persists that these established ethical criteria are too naïvely utilitarian. Nonetheless, a sensible approach would be to appreciate the merits of ethical criteria for screening whilst remaining alert to the need to balance the benefits of less than perfect screening with the urge to be ethically pristine, and to balance a utilitarian approach to screening ethics with other important perspectives.

Benefit

The discussion could go in various directions at this point. We might focus on one particularly contentious health screening programme and discuss in depth its merits and ethical status. Should American citizens undergo mental health screening (Lenzer 2004) or screening for obesity

(US Preventive Services Task Force 2003)? Should we screen for an adult-onset or late-onset genetic disorder such as Huntington's disease? Alternatively, and more broadly, it would be useful to juxtapose screening programmes of the same kind that contrast in ways that tease out our intuitions and principles. For example, one might juxtapose different genetic screening programmes, or different mental health-related programmes. There is only space in the rest of this chapter to pursue one such strategy, by exploring a contemporary ethical theme that runs through discussions of various proposed health screening programmes. A good candidate is compulsory screening and informed choice (Gostin 2000: 192ff; Childress et al. 2002: 173ff.; Jepson et al. 2005), but since this is very close to the topic of compulsory vaccination discussed in the previous chapter, here we take up the theme of benefit.

The basic problem

There is a basic problem about the benefit of screening. To explain, consider screening that is on safe moral ground. Morally uncontentious health screening meets the kinds of criteria discussed above, such as that the screened-for condition is important, its epidemiology and detection are uncontentious, and so on. The current neonatal screening programme for PKU seems like a paradigmatic case. An important member of the list of criteria met by such morally pristine programmes concerns benefit. Intuitively, it seems plausible that a necessary condition for developing a screening programme is that it produces benefit. Even at this stage the criterion requires clarifications, such as that the benefit should outweigh harms, as stated in number 15 of the NSC's criteria, above. Nonetheless, an uncontentious starting point is that a screening programme is not ethical unless it produces substantial benefit.

Benefit to whom and of what kind? A two-part ethical criterion suggests itself. First, the screening programme should benefit the screenees. Second, the benefit to screenees is earlier, more effective medical interventions to treat the screened-for condition. Let's call this complex condition the 'benefit criterion'. It tallies with our standard case of an ethically pristine screening programme: babies found to have PKU benefit, and they do so by receiving earlier, so more effective, treatments that ameliorate their condition. So far, so good. However, there are feasible new screening programmes – genetic screening programmes, most notably – that sound very worthwhile, but which evidently fail to meet the benefit criterion. This raises the basic problem about benefit and screening. If we insist on the benefit criterion then apparently worthwhile, feasible screening programmes would be ruled out. But if, on the other hand, we do not insist that programmes meet the benefit criterion, then how far, and on what grounds, should we go in allowing programmes that do not enable true positives to receive earlier, so more effective, medical treatments?

The key to a proper discussion of this problem is to be very clear about the two parts of the benefit criterion, namely, who benefits from a screening programme, and the kind of benefit the programme offers. It is difficult to keep them apart because they are so intimately related. For example, the most common situation in which we consider screening for a condition that does not benefit the screenee is where there is no cure for, or effective medical treatment of, the screened-for condition, but there are other kinds of benefits to other people. But we must keep these aspects apart because, though intimately connected, they raise different issues in which different considerations arise. So, one question is about whether we are justified in screening people, not because they will benefit, but because others will. Another related but distinct question is about whether we are justified in screening people in order to provide benefits other than in the form of earlier, so more effective, medical interventions. Bearing this in mind, let's consider some instructive cases.

Expanding the benefit criterion: newborn screening for MRDD and autism

Bailey et al. (2005) discuss newborn screening for development disabilities. The premise of their argument is that '[h]istorically, the decision to screen a newborn has been a conservative one' (p. 1891) because it is based on the concept of presumptive benefit. In fact, the established criterion for newborn screening they discern is the benefit criterion defined above: early detection of the condition allows for medical treatment that benefits the child by altering the course of the disease. But when Bailey et al. looked at the newly feasible screening programme for mental retardation and developmental disability (MRDD), they found that it fails to meet the benefit criterion because there is no cure or medical treatment for the condition. Nonetheless, the programme would produce great benefit to the child (though not in the form of a cure or other medical intervention that can alter the course of the condition), their family, and society at large. The authors conclude that the case of MRDD suggests that we should 'reframe' – i.e., expand – the concept of presumptive benefit at work in newborn screening to allow such programmes (cf. Gray 2004).

Let's look more closely at the three main categories of beneficiaries of MRDD screening Bailey et al. discuss, i.e., true positives, their families, and society. Concerning the first, despite the facts that MRDD is not curable, and that much more research is required, it seems clear that 'early intervention programmes can positively influence the development and behaviour of many young children with [these] disabilities' (p. 1891). Second, families of true positives benefit in various ways: 'early intervention can enhance the parents' capacity to care for and teach their child, build advocacy skills, promote an optimistic view of the future, improve family quality of life, reduce stress, and enhance formal and informal supports' (p. 1890). And, thirdly, an MRDD screening programme would provide various societal benefits. These are mainly research oriented, including improving epidemiological data and aetiological understanding of the condition, promoting research and development relevant to the condition, and improving tests for treatment efficacy (cf. Eide 1997).

Let's narrow the lens even more, and focus in on the benefits to true positives. It is important to bear in mind here the ways that early interventions are traditionally seen to benefit true positives, namely, curing the disease, altering its course and ameliorating its effects. Medical treatment can neither cure nor alter the course of MRDD; but other kinds of interventions more effectively benefit children with the condition because of earlier detection. Furthermore, it seems clear that what are categorized as benefits to people other than the screenees are also of indirect benefit to the screenees. For example, many of the benefits characterized by Bailey et al. as benefits to families will have knock-on effects that enhance the quality of the true positive's life ('early intervention can enhance the parents' capacity to care for and teach their child ... reduce stress' and so on). Arguably, even societal benefits are of indirect benefit to screenees in the sense that future generations of people with the condition in question will be helped by the research undertakings the authors mention.

The fact that MRDD screening would provide such benefits to true positives, families and society indicates that, at least so far as benefit is concerned, the programme is justified; hence, Bailey et al. conclude that we should relax or reframe the notion of benefit that figures in discussions of newborn screening. Autism is a similar case. It, too, is a condition which might seem to fall outside the original standard for newborn screening as Bailey et al. interpret it, since medicine can neither cure nor alter the course of the condition (Strock 2004). Until recently, autism screening centred on behavioural markers for autism: notably, the Checklist for Autism in Toddlers (Baron-Cohen et al. 1996); the Modified CHAT (Robins et al. 2001); the Screening Tool for Autism in Two-year olds (Stone et al. 2000, 2004); and the Social Communication Questionnaire (Berument et al. 1999; cf. Eaves et al. 2006). Screening for behavioural markers can be administered only after the child is old enough to display the relevant behaviour traits, which is not as early as would be most beneficial (Santangelo and Tsatsanis 2005; cf. Zwaigenbaum et al. 2005). An exciting development involves looking for biological (as opposed to behavioural) markers for autism, which can be detected much earlier. For example, it has been suggested that a simple neonatal blood spot to test for autism might be developed on the basis of identifiable features of the blood of autistic people, which would enable much earlier detection (Amaral et al. 2005; see, also, Nelson et al. 2001).

The case for newborn screening for autism by blood spot seems very similar to MRDD screening: despite there being no medical cure or way of medically altering the course of the disease, the programme is justified because it promises other benefits, both direct and indirect, to true positives, as well as independent benefits to families and society. What makes both programmes relatively uncontentious is how beneficial they would be, both directly and indirectly, to the true positives. The fact that the programme would independently benefit others in other ways only serves to confirm the programme's acceptability. So, we should 'reframe' the notion of presumptive benefit at work in newborn screening to allow these programmes.

The difficulty is that this very cogent argument for relaxing and reframing the notion of presumptive benefit creates two slippery slopes. This is where we need to bear in mind the two parts of the benefit criterion distinguished above, i.e., that the screening programme benefits the true positives, and benefits them in the form of earlier, more effective treatments. The first slippery slope is about who benefits: once we take other people into account, are we on a slippery slope to allowing screening programmes that do not benefit – or, indeed, are actually detrimental to – true positives? The second slippery slope is about what kinds of benefits programmes provide: once we take other benefits into account, are we on a slippery slope to allowing screening programmes that do not even aim to enable more effective treatment, but which have quite different, arguably non-medical, objectives? Both slippery slopes might sound fanciful. One might think that, surely, all health screening offers medical benefits to screenees, whatever other benefits to other people are on offer. But there are good examples of programmes that threaten to take us down both the slippery slopes just described.

First slippery slope: screening to the detriment of true positives

The clearest examples of screening programmes that might not only fail to benefit, but actually be to the detriment of, true positives are antenatal screening programmes. The obvious thought here is that true positives do not benefit from some programmes because the typical upshot of a positive result is the termination of the pregnancy. This is what fuelled the debate about whether genetic counselling is, can be, or should be, non-directive (Clarke 1991, 1998; Michie et al. 1998; Bartels et al. 1997). Most starkly, it has been suggested that success in genetic counselling should be measured by the number of terminations of pregnancy it results in (Chadwick 1993). The general consensus is against such an outcome measure; nonetheless, the proposal demonstrates the relationship between antenatal screening and abortion.

There are numerous complications here. First, we have to distinguish two kinds of cases of antenatal abnormalities, which Glover (2001) calls 'disastrous' and 'moderately severe' disability. Although the distinction is vague, clear examples of the former include conditions such as Tay–Sachs and trisomy 18, i.e., conditions that would make the child's life 'less than one worth living'. The range of moderately severe disabilities includes conditions that give rise to mild forms of physical and learning disability, such as Down's syndrome and less severe spina bifida. Arguably, the termination of a pregnancy that would result in the former kind of disability is a benefit to true positives. Can the same be said of antenatal screening for clear cases of moderately severe disability?

Let's focus the discussion on whether true positives benefit from the detection of conditions such as Down's syndrome (National Screening Committee 2002; Camilleri-Ferrante 2000). Again, there are complications and caveats. For one thing, it is certainly not the case that all parents would terminate a pregnancy because their child would have Down's syndrome. Note, too, that if the pregnancy does continue, indirect benefits of the kind mentioned in the context of MRDD and autism screening would accrue to true positives: i.e., the child would benefit because parents would be better able to adjust to the condition of their baby, prepare other family members, access services more quickly, etc. But, such points notwithstanding, it is clear that an assumption underlying the Down's syndrome screening programme is that many parents of true positives will decide to terminate the pregnancy. And in fact many parents do terminate the pregnancy given a positive result. So, it is surely fair to describe the programme as at least in part a public health endeavour designed to reduce the birth prevalence of a chromosomal disorder.

The Kantian argument

To see the moral problem here we need to recall some moral theory from Part I. Deontology is the view that some actions are by their very nature right or wrong (Chapter 2). One Kantian version of this view is that actions which treat people as mere means to ends, as opposed to ends-in-themselves, are wrong in principle. Arguably, the Down's syndrome screening programme is a case in point: disabled people are being used as mere means to an end, namely, the public health goal of reducing the birth prevalence of a chromosomal disorder.

How strong is the Kantian objection to screening for foetal abnormalities such as Down's syndrome (Reynolds 2003)? One retort is that such screening programmes do not turn true positives into mere means, because the screenee is in fact the mother, not the foetus. The idea here is that the screened population comprises pregnant women, the point of antenatal screening programmes being to determine how their pregnancy is developing. But is this convincing? Because Down's syndrome is a chromosomal disorder, it is clear who has it: the foetus, not the woman. So, it seems equally clear that the screened population is made up of foetuses, the true positives being the ones correctly identified as having the condition.

Suppose we accept that the screenees are the scanned and tested foetuses. Still, we can question whether the programme turns them into the mere means to achieve public health goals. A somewhat technical rejoinder is to argue that people with Down's syndrome are not 'persons' in the specific sense in which this term is used in Kantian ethics; i.e., they lack the capacities and characteristics that make a human being a person. This is not a matter of being derogatory towards people with Down's syndrome; the point is simply that Kant ruled out treating persons as mere means, and, arguably, Down's syndrome people fail to meet the conditions for personhood. But this is unconvincing. For one thing, many Down's syndrome people do meet standard criteria for personhood, such as a capacity for rationality, language-use, self-consciousness, and so on, because their learning disability is relatively moderate. Besides, the Kantian can avoid this manoeuvre by simply changing the example from antenatal screening for Down's syndrome to some other moderately serious physical disability that leaves the individual's psychological capacities, and hence their personhood, intact.

Another tack is to argue that an adult with a moderately severe disability such as Down's syndrome is a person in the Kantian sense, but the foetuses that are said to be sacrificed for the sake of public health objectives are not. This would be based on the fact that the foetus is at best a potential person as opposed to an actual person. This is a very complex area, and not one to go deeply into here (Tooley 1998). It will suffice to map out the options. One view is that potential persons lack the moral status of persons, so we can do what we like with and to them. This is too extreme: none of us started to acquire the characteristics of personhood until we were about two years old, so, on this extreme view, we can do what we like with, and to, an infant (Tooley 1972). Another view is that life, and with it high moral status, starts at conception. The problem with this is that there are cogent arguments to the conclusion that, up to about 14 days when gastrulation takes place, a pre-embryo exists that cannot be one and the same as the resultant person because, for example, it has the ability to twin (Munthe 2001). In between these two rather extreme views is gradualism: moral status increases as the human individual develops. Arguably, the fact that the gradualist view is appealing counts in favour of the Kantian proscription on antenatal screening for moderately severe disabilities because therapeutic abortions undertaken on medical grounds are permitted relatively late in a pregnancy, when the human being has acquired a good deal of moral status.

So, the Kantian objection to antenatal screening for moderate disabilities such as Down's syndrome seems quite robust. It is worth noting that it fuels criticism from the community of disabled commentators on medical ethics, who press certain rather troubling questions about antenatal screening programmes. Why try to screen out of society conditions that, though not inconsiderable, leave one with a physical disability and a very worthwhile life? Specifically, what does such an agenda say about societal attitudes towards disabilities and the disabled? A focus of the debate here is on how feasible it is to use antenatal screening and termination to combat a disability, on the one hand, whilst maintaining a positive societal attitude towards extant disabled people, on the other (Parens and Asch 1999, 2000; Gillott 2001; Herissone-Kelly 2003).

The important point for present purposes is not to decide whether we are justified in screening for conditions such as Down's syndrome, let alone which of the various possible programmes is optimal (Serra-Prat et al. 1998). Rather, the central point concerns the ethical requirement on screening programmes to benefit true positives. The cases of MRDD and autism screening suggest that, if we make the criterion for ethical screening too narrow by insisting that screening benefits true positives in the form of early medical treatment, then we rule out very worthwhile programmes. So, we should relax or reframe the benefit criterion. But the case of antenatal screening for Down's syndrome illustrates the danger of a slippery slope towards relaxing the criterion too far. Arguably, Down's syndrome screening is unethical on the Kantian grounds that, far from benefiting true positives, it threatens to turn them into mere means to the public health objective of reducing the birth prevalence of a chromosomal disorder, as opposed to ends-in-themselves.

Second slippery slope: screening for the sake of non-medical benefits

There is a second slippery slope to consider. This concerns the other part of the benefit criterion, i.e., the kind of benefit health screening should provide. Recall the paradigm: ethical screening provides benefits other than in the form of medical cures or treatments that alter the course of a disease. Cases such as MRDD and autism screening suggest that we should relax this to allow other kinds of benefits. Does this put us on a slippery slope towards screening for the sake of non-medical benefits?

One way of pursuing this question focuses on information; screening for information has become an important case study of a screening benefit that is not – at least, not directly – medical. Let's distinguish three kinds of cases in which one might screen for information: first, screening for information that allows true positives to make lifestyle changes that can help to protect or improve their health; second, screening for information about conditions which true positives can do nothing to avoid; and third, screening for information that increases reproductive choice. The US Preventive Services Task Force's recommendation that clinicians screen all adult patients for obesity, mentioned above, is an example of the first kind of programme. Genetic screening for adult-onset or late-onset Huntington's disease is an example of the second category. And mass population screening for cystic fibrosis (CF) carrier status is an example of the third. Each of these has generated much discussion and an extensive literature (Slevin 2004; Duncan et al. 2005; Massie et al. 2005). Let's take each in turn.

Given that obesity is a risk factor for heart and other diseases, the US Preventive Services Task Force's recommendation to screen for obesity seems justifiable because information about BMI might benefit true positives in terms of disease prevention. Of course, there is a myriad of questions raised by the recommendation. Some are about the details of the programme. For example, the US Preventive Services Task Force (2003) concluded that 'the benefits of screening and behavioral interventions outweigh potential harms' despite admitting that '[n]o evidence was found that addressed the harms of counseling and behavioral interventions'. Other questions recall the discussion of behaviour modification in Chapter 7. How far is it permissible to go on influencing behaviours in the name of health gain; does the US Preventive Services Task Force's recommendation amount to a policy of 'naming and shaming' or something more worthy? Nonetheless, at least we can say that the programme meets the benefit criterion for ethical screening insofar as it is effective in preventing disease.

Huntington's disease is an example of the second kind of case in which one might screen for information, distinguished above, i.e., screening for information about conditions which true positives can do nothing to avoid. Arguably, on the grounds that Huntington's disease is neither avoidable by dint of lifestyle choices, nor currently treatable, being informed of a genetic predisposition to its onset would provide nothing but harm in the form of depression, anxiety, etc.: 'The technology to offer predisposition to genetic testing for many late-onset disorders is rapidly becoming available, yet how one uses this technology to benefit patients is not always clear' (McKinnon et al. 1997). Added to this are the well-documented worries about consent and confidentiality that the detection of such a condition creates (Visintainer et al. 2001).

But we should pause for reflection here because many commentators argue that predictive testing for adult-onset genetic conditions would benefit true positives. In fact, Bailey et al.'s (2005) point, discussed above, that the notion of benefit at work in newborn screening is too narrow and conservative, has been made in precisely this context: 'the claim that there are no benefits from early testing is based on an unjustifiably narrow view of benefits that ignores significant advantages that testing actually provides' (Rhodes 2006: 609; cf. Burke et al. 2001). How might information about a predisposition to Huntington's disease benefit a true positive? Some people might well live a different, more fulfilling life in the knowledge that a cogent ripe old age is, for them, unlikely. Some might feel empowered to make more of their youth and middle age. Conversely, reacting to the unanticipated onset of a genetic disorder such as Huntington's disease with outrage at having made what turn out to be inappropriate lifestyle choices is surely understandable. This recalls the discussion of the contested nature of health (and other, related concepts such as illness and disease) in Chapter 6. On a narrow, negative view of health as the absence of disease, screening for genetic information about risk of late-onset disorders is just irrelevant because the disease is not treatable; but on a broader, more positive account of health as well-being, such a programme might well, at least in some cases, be health promoting.

Now let's consider an example of the third kind of case in which one might screen for information, i.e., screening for information that increases reproductive choice, by focusing on mass population genetic screening for CF carrier status. The central concern about this is neatly captured by Stone and Stewart (1996: 4):

> The 'information' aim [of CF screening] ... is qualitatively different from that of most other forms of screening in that it encapsulates no preventive principle (except in a most tenuous and indirect fashion). Instead, the generation of information is regarded as a worthwhile aim in itself, regardless of outcome. This represents a paradigm shift in the philosophy of screening and deserves closer scrutiny.

Stone and Stewart report a prevailing orthodoxy that population screening for genetic carrier states is a good thing. They dissent from this view by questioning both the assumption that the information is beneficial to individuals, and the presumption that a 'right to know' grounds screening for genetic information.

We should follow Stone and Stewart's lead and put the screening benefit of information under closer scrutiny. A principal benefit of information gained from such screening is increased reproductive choice. Whatever else might count against it, here, at least, is one sense in which mass population screening for CF seems justifiable in terms of the informational benefits to be gained. This is best demonstrated by contrasting it with two other programmes that have figured prominently in the discussions in this chapter, namely, screening for obesity and Down's syndrome. To take each in turn, first, the great benefit of obesity screening is that, at least indirectly, it can contribute to the worthwhile public health goal of preventing important prevalent diseases, by providing the information to ground lifestyle and other changes. Likewise, carrier status screening for CF would allow couples to avoid having CF children, thereby reducing the birth prevalence of

CF. So, screening for CF seems *prima facie* justified on the same grounds as screening for obesity.

Now contrast carrier status screening for CF with Down's syndrome screening. The Kantian argument against the latter is that extant true positives (existing foetuses with the chromosomal disorder) are turned into mere means of achieving a public health goal (reduced birth prevalence of Down's syndrome). But, at least in some kinds of CF screening programmes – i.e., those in which the couple are screened pre-conception – arguably, there are no extant CF sufferers to be turned into mere means. Specifically, on the basis of the genetic information acquired by the programme, a couple might decide against starting a family, or use donor gametes that are free of the genetic fault. In both cases, the public health goal of reducing the birth prevalence of CF is achieved without using anyone as a mere means: it is not the case that CF children are substituted by healthy ones, because the former never exist in the first place. Hence the Kantian argument, seemingly powerful against Down's syndrome screening, simply does not get hold in the case of screening for CF. This is a major point in favour of the view that pre-conception genetic screening is morally superior to antenatal screening.

Concluding remarks

This chapter has discussed the ethical dimension in screening. First, the nature of screening, and current and proposed screening programmes, were described. The second part of the chapter considered issues that apply to health screening in general, including worries about, and putative general ethical principles or criteria to be met by, all screening programmes. The third part illustrates the ethical dimension of health screening by focusing on the theme of benefit. Here, two slippery slopes were discerned. The first is a slippery slope towards screening to the detriment of true positives. The Kantian argument that antenatal Down's syndrome screening is ethically dubious because it turns true positives into mere means was used to illustrate this. The second slippery slope is towards screening for the sake of non-medical benefits. Screening for information was discussed as a case in point. Clearly, there is much more to be said, both about the specific screening programmes mentioned in this chapter and about screening in general. Nonetheless, a framework for the ethical analysis of screening programmes has been introduced.

Concluding Remarks |

The aim of this book has been to engage in a fairly wide-ranging discussion of public health ethics, as opposed to developing a narrow thesis. Given this, a conclusion summing up the book's position would not be appropriate. Instead, it will better to comment on two themes that have run through the text.

The re-description problem

The first theme comprises an interesting and challenging problem that arose at numerous points in the foregoing. For the sake of a label, this can be called the re-description problem. To explain the problem we need to recall, from the Introduction, the central dilemma in public health ethics, i.e., between the rights and freedoms of individuals, and the needs and good of the community. The re-description problem is that what seem like fruitful discussions of the ethics of specific public health activities end up merely re-describing that central dilemma, albeit in novel terms. Some illustrations of this problem from the main text of this book might help to clarify it.

An early example of the re-description problem arose in the discussion of rights and public health in the Introduction. The point was made there that the appeal to rights in public health ethics is likely to merely restate the central dilemma between individuals and communities. This is because the central dilemma can be put in terms of rights: we are in a quandary about whether to prioritize the rights of the individual or communal rights. Another case in point arose in Chapter 4 where the appeal to the communitarian critique of liberal individualism was discussed. It was argued there that the appeal is relatively uncompelling because it threatens to merely re-describe the central dilemma in public health ethics – i.e., between the individual and the community – in political-philosophical terms.

Further illustrations can be taken from Part II of the book. For example, the harm principle figures prominently in the discussions of the ethics of behaviour modification in Chapter 7 and the ethics of mass immunization programmes in Chapter 9. But quite what the harm principle is, how it applies in such contexts, and how powerful a consideration it provides in ethical debates are contestable. Crucially, there is the danger that the contest over these will merely re-describe the central public health ethics dilemma. For example, those who want to prioritize communal benefits over individual rights will define and apply the harm principle in a way that justifies aggressive behaviour modification programmes and compulsory immunization policies. Opponents who want to prioritize individual rights over communal benefits will contest the proffered definition and/or application of the harm principle in order to resist such programmes and policies.

The problem is that what looks like fruitful debate is in danger of collapsing into a mere re-description of the central dilemma between individuals and communities, albeit in increasingly highbrow terms. This re-description problem is a serious challenge to public health ethicists. But it is not insurmountable. Nor should it be exaggerated. For one thing, not all debates in public health ethics are mere re-descriptions of the central dilemma. Progress in some areas is feasible. It depends on the problem at hand and the considerations that can be brought to bear. In very many of the discussions reported in Part II, progress was made by clarifying the problem, and by distinguishing, defining and applying relevant theoretical and practical considerations. So, whilst it is worth making the rather subtle re-description problem explicit, it does not rule out progress in public health ethics.

Public health ethics and philosophy

A second theme worth remarking on in this conclusion concerns the relationship between academic philosophy and public health. The background to this is Nijhuis and van der Maesen's (1994) invitation to debate the philosophical foundations of public health:

> most theoretical debates about the pros and cons of public health approaches are confined to the methodological scientific level. Philosophical foundations such as underlying ontological notions are rarely part of public health discussions, but these are always implicit and lie behind the arguments and reasoning of different viewpoints or traditions. (P. 1)

Nijhuis and van der Maesen's short piece was important in bringing the philosophical underpinnings of public health to attention. Their 'invitation' stimulated a number of subsequent published works on the theme (Tatara 2002; Weed 1999; van der Maesen and Nijhuis 2000; D.E. Beauchamp 1995; cf. Thomasma 1997). Generally speaking, it motivated the increasing interest in public health in the philosophical community.

How does academic philosophy inform public health ethics? One way is very general and stylistic. Public health ethics problems are complex and involve numerous concepts, arguments and points of view. They are also very emotive; the point was made at the very start of this book that medicine and health care, including public health, deal with urgent aspects of people's lives. These features make the subject matter of public health ethics appealing to writers and commentators. But they also make certain intellectual virtues necessary if debates are to be properly prosecuted. Specifically, public health activities should be debated with conceptual clarity, argumentative rigour and expressive precision. These are the trade-marks of (academic, analytic) philosophy. So, public health ethics can benefit from acquiring philosophers' intellectual habits. Of course, analytic philosophy is not to everyone's taste, and there are innumerable other perspectives from which to view public health dilemmas: feminism, the ethics of care, Marxism, post-structuralism, post-colonialism, and so on. Nonetheless, the precision and argumentative rigour typical of academic philosophy is to be recommended, and, crucially, it is in no way inimical to these other perspectives.

More specifically, public health ethics can and should be informed by theories developed in moral and political philosophy. A number of theoretical perspectives on public health ethics problems were introduced in Part I, including consequentialist and non-consequentialist rejoinders to naïve utilitarianism in public health, and, from political philosophy, the liberal objection and its rejoinders. To reiterate a point made at the end of Part I, it would be a mistake to conclude from the plethora of theories discussed and applied in this book that anything goes in public health because almost any intervention can be justified by some theory or other. Public health ethics is not the game of finding some theoretical basis for what one wants to do, nor is an intervention properly justified because it has some small degree of theoretical support. An intervention might enjoy *prima facie* support from certain moral and political theories that is overridden by other considerations; on the other hand, properly justified public health activities will enjoy strong theoretical support. To discern which interventions enjoy such support requires knowledge, and the proper application, of moral theory and political philosophy.

Finally, many of the specific issues debated in this book are rooted in parts of philosophy other than moral and political theory. For example, it is impossible to get to grips with epidemiological ethics without asking questions rooted in the philosophy of science about, for example, causation and underdetermination. This was stressed in Chapter 5 where theoretical challenges to epidemiology were discussed. Another good example is the analysis of health concepts. As discussed in Chapter 6, clarifying the nature of health is crucial to the justification of public health interventions in general, and health promotion activities in particular. An understandable reaction to such philosophical musings is that they start too far back: i.e., they are too academic for such a practical endeavour as public health. But the point was made in Chapter 6 that, although conceptual questions – in that case, about the nature of health – might seem merely academic, this is a mistake because conceptual conclusions have practical effects. In fact, one of the things that make public health ethics such an interesting subject is that, apart from its practical importance, it engages with deep philosophical questions.

References

Aldridge, M.A. 2012: Addressing non-adherence to antipsychotic medication: a harm-reduction approach. *Journal of Psychiatric and Mental Health Nursing*, 19, 85–96.

Amaral, D.G., Corbett, B., Kantor, A., Becker, C., Kakkanaiah, V., Deng, J., Bacalman, S. and Schulman, H. 2005: Immunophenotyping and proteomic and metabolomic profiling of children with autism. In *Program and Abstracts of the 4th International Meeting for Autism Research* (May 5–7, 2005; Boston, MA).

American College of Epidemiology 2000: Ethics guidelines. *Annals of Epidemiology*, 10 (8), 487–97.

Anand, S., Fabienne, P. and Sen, A. (eds) 2004: *Public Health, Ethics and Equality*. Oxford: Oxford University Press.

Andreasen, A.R. (ed.) 2001: *Ethics in Social Marketing*. Washington, DC: Georgetown University Press.

Annas, G.J. 2002: Bioterrorism, public health, and civil liberties. *The New England Journal of Medicine*, 346 (17), 1337–42.

Appell, D. 2001: The new uncertainty principle. *Scientific American*, January, 18–19.

Applegate, J. 2000: The precautionary preference: an American perspective on the precautionary principle. *Human and Ecological Risk Assessment*, 6 (3), 413–43.

Ashcroft, R.E. 2011: Personal financial incentives in health promotion: where do they fit in an ethic of autonomy? *Health Expectations*, 14, 191–200.

Austoker, J. 1999: Gaining informed consent for screening. *British Medical Journal*, 319 (7212), 722–3.

Avineri, S. and de-Shalit, A. (eds) 1992: *Communitarianism and Individualism*. Oxford: Oxford University Press.

Bailey, D.B., Skinner, D. and Warren, S.F. 2005: Newborn screening for developmental disabilities: reframing presumptive benefit. *American Journal of Public Health*, 95 (11), 1889–93.

Barbor, T.F. 1990: Epidemiology, advocacy and ideology in alcohol studies. *Journal of Studies on Alcohol*, 51 (4), 293–5.

Baron-Cohen, S., Cox, A., Baird, G., Swettenham, J., Nightingale, N., Morgan, K., Drew, A. and Charman, T. 1996: Psychological markers in the detection of autism in infancy in a large population. *The British Journal of Psychiatry*, 168 (2), 158–63.

Bartels, D.M., LeRoy, B.S., McCarthy, P. and Caplan, A.L. 1997: Nondirectiveness in genetic counselling: a survey of practitioners. *American Journal of Medical Genetics*, 72 (2), 172–9.

Bayer, R. 1981: Voluntary health risks and public policy: Introduction. *Hastings Center Report*, 11 (5), 26.

Bayer, R. and Fairchild, A.L. 2004: The genesis of public health ethics. *Bioethics*, 18 (6), 473–92.

Bayer, R., Dubler, N.N. and Landesman, S. 1993: The dual epidemic of tuberculosis and AIDS: ethical and policy issues in screening and treatment. *American Journal of Public Health*, 83 (5), 649–54.

Bayer, R., Gostin, L., Javitt, G. and Brandt, A. 2002: Tobacco advertising in the United States: a proposal for a constitutionally acceptable form of regulation. *Journal of the American Medical Association*, 287 (22), 2990–5.

Bayley, C. 1995: Our world views (may be) incommensurable: now what? *The Journal of Medicine and Philosophy*, 20 (3), 271–84.

Beauchamp, D.E. 1980: Public health and individual liberty. *Annual Review of Public Health*, 1, 121–36.

Beauchamp, D.E. 1985: Community: the neglected tradition of public health. *Hastings Center Report*, 15 (6), 28–36.

Beauchamp, D.E. 1988: *The Health of the Republic: Epidemics, Medicine, and Moralism as Challenges to Democracy*. Philadelphia, PA: Temple University Press.

Beauchamp, D.E. 1995: III. Philosophy of public health. In W.T. Reich (editor-in-chief) *Encyclopedia of Bioethics* (revised edn) (Vol. 4). New York: Simon & Schuster Macmillan, 2161–6.

Beauchamp, D.E. and Steinbock, B. (eds) 1999: *New Ethics for the Public's Health*. Oxford: Oxford University Press.

Beauchamp, T.L. 1995: Principlism and its alleged competitors. *Kennedy Institute of Ethics Journal*, 5 (3), 181–98.

Beauchamp, T.L. 1996: Moral foundations. In S.S. Coughlin and T.L. Beauchamp (eds) *Ethics and Epidemiology*. Oxford: Oxford University Press, 24–51.

244   References

Beauchamp, T.L. and Childress, J.F. 2013: *Principles of Biomedical Ethics* (7th edn). Oxford: Oxford University Press.

Beauchamp, T.L., Cook, R.R., Fayerweather, W.E., Raabe, G.K., Thar, W.E., Cowles, S.R. and Spivey, G.H. 1991: Ethical guidelines for epidemiologists. *Journal of Clinical Epidemiology*, 44 (suppl. 1), 151–69.

Becker, G. and Murphy, K.M. 1988: A theory of rational addiction. *Journal of Political Economy*, 96 (4), 675–700.

Beirness, D.J., Jesseman, R., Notarandrea, R. and Perron, M. 2008: *Harm Reduction: What's in a Name?* Ottawa: Canadian Centre on Substance Abuse. Available at http://www.canadianharmreduction.com/node/1077 (accessed September 2013).

Bell, D. 2012: Communitarianism. In E.N. Zalta (ed.) *The Stanford Encyclopedia of Philosophy*. Available at http://plato.stanford.edu/entries/communitarianism/ (accessed March 2014).

Bellaby, P. 2003: Communication and miscommunication of risk: understanding UK parents' attitudes to combined MMR vaccination. *British Medical Journal*, 327 (7417), 725–8.

Berlin, I. 1969: Two concepts of liberty. In *Four Essays on Liberty*. Oxford: Oxford University Press, 118–72.

Berument, S.K., Rutter, M., Lord, C., Pickles, A. and Bailey, A. 1999: Autism screening questionnaire: diagnostic validity. *The British Journal of Psychiatry*, 175 (5), 444–51.

Boorse, C. 1975: On the distinction between disease and illness. *Philosophy and Public Affairs*, 5 (1), 49–68.

Boorse, C. 1977: Health as a theoretical concept. *Philosophy of Science*, 44 (4), 542–73.

Boorse, C. 1997: A rebuttal on health. In J.M. Humber and R.F. Almeder (eds) *What is Disease?* Totowa, NJ: Humana Press, 3–134.

Bradley, P. 2000: Should childhood immunisation be compulsory? In P. Bradley and A. Burls (eds) *Ethics in Public and Community Health*. London: Routledge, 167–76.

Bradley, P. and Burls, A. 2000: *Ethics in Public and Community Health*. New York: Routledge.

Brecher, B. 1999: Liberal and communitarian conceptions of medical need, with particular reference to the management of organ transplantation. *Archives of Hellenic Medicine*, 16 (6), 609–14.

Brennan, P. and Croft, P. 1994: Interpreting the results of observational research: chance is not such a fine thing. *British Medical Journal*, 309 (6956), 727–30.

British Medical Association 2003: *Childhood Immunisation: A Guide for Healthcare Professionals*. London: British Medical Association.

British Medical Association 2005: *Population Genetic Screening and Testing: A Briefing on Current Programmes and Technologies*. London: British Medical Association.

Buchanan, A., Brock, D., Daniels, N. and Wikler, D. 2000: *From Chance to Choice: Genetics and Justice*. Cambridge: Cambridge University Press.

Buchanan, D., Khoshnood, K., Stopka, T., Shaw, S., Santelices, C. and Singer, M. 2002: Ethical dilemmas created by the criminalization of status behaviors: case examples from ethnographic field research with injection drug users. *Health Education and Behavior*, 29 (1), 30–42.

Buchanan, D.R. 2000: *An Ethic for Health Promotion. Rethinking the Sources of Human Well-Being.* Oxford: Oxford University Press.

Buchanan, I. 1995: The purpose–process gap in health promotion. In D. Seedhouse (ed.) *Reforming Health Care: The Philosophy and Practice of International Health Reform.* Chichester: John Wiley & Sons, 221–7.

Budetti, P. 2001: Personal freedom or public health? (2). In M. Marinker (ed.) *Medicine and Humanity.* London: King's Fund, 71–85.

Burke, W., Coughlin, S.S., Lee, N.C., Weed, D.L. and Khoury, M.J. 2001: Application of population screening principles to genetic screening for adult-onset conditions. *Genetic Testing*, 5 (3), 201–11.

Buttiglione, R. and Pasquini, M. 2002: The challenge of government in the constructing of health care policy. In P. Taboada, K.F. Cuddeback and P. Donohue-White (eds) *Person, Society and Value: Towards a Personalist Concept of Health.* Dordrecht: Kluwer, 229–40.

Cadman, D., Chambers, L., Feldman, W. and Sackett, D. 1984: Assessing the effectiveness of community screening programs. *Journal of the American Medical Association*, 251 (12), 1580–5.

Calandrillo, S. 2004: Vanishing vaccinations: why are so many Americans opting out of vaccinating their children? *University of Michigan Journal of Law Reform*, 37 (2), 353–440.

Callahan, D. 1984: Autonomy: a moral good, not a moral obsession. *Hastings Center Report*, 14 (5), 40–2.

Callahan, D. (ed.) 2000: *Promoting Healthy Behaviour: How Much Freedom? Whose Responsibility?* Washington, DC: Georgetown University Press.

Callahan, D. and Jennings, B. 2002: Ethics and public health: forging a strong relationship. *American Journal of Public Health*, 92 (2), 169–76.

Calman, K.C. and Downie, R.S. 2002: Ethical principles and ethical issues in public health. In R. Detels, J. McEwen, R. Beaglehole and H. Tanaka (eds) *Oxford Textbook of Public Health* (4th edn). Oxford: Oxford University Press, 387–99.

Calnan, M. 1987: *Health and Illness: The Lay Perspective.* London: Tavistock.

Camilleri-Ferrante, C. 2000: Antenatal screening. In P. Bradley and A. Burls (eds) *Ethics in Public and Community Health.* New York: Routledge, 106–18.

Campbell, A.V. 1990: Education or indoctrination? The issue of autonomy in health education. In S. Doxiadis (ed.) *Ethics in Health Education.* Chichester: John Wiley & Sons, 15–27.

Caney, S. 1992: Liberalism and communitarianism: a misconceived debate? *Political Studies*, XL, 273–89.

Cappelen, A.W. and Norheim, O.F. 2005: Responsibility in health care: a liberal egalitarian approach. *Journal of Medical Ethics*, 31 (8), 476–80.

Capron, A. 1991: Protection of research subjects: do special rules apply in epidemiology? *Journal of Clinical Epidemiology*, 44 (suppl. 1), 81–9.

Chadwick, R. 1993: What counts as success in genetic counselling? *Journal of Medical Ethics*, 19 (1), 43–6.

Chadwick, R. and Levitt, M. (eds) 1998: *Ethical Issues in Community Health Care*. London: Arnold.

Chaloner, C. 2003: Confidentiality. In S. Holland (ed.) *Introducing Nursing Ethics: Themes in Theory and Practice*. Wiltshire: APS, 65–90.

Charlton, B.G. 1993: Public health and medicine – a different kind of ethics? *Journal of the Royal Society of Medicine*, 86 (4), 194–5.

Charlton, B.G. 2001: Personal freedom or public health? (1). In M. Marinker (ed.) *Medicine and Humanity*. London: King's Fund, 55–69.

Childress, J.F. and Bernheim, R.G. 2003: Beyond the liberal and communitarian impasse: a framework and vision for public health. *Florida Law Review*, 55 (5), 1191–219.

Childress, J.F., Faden, R.R., Gaare, R.D., Gostin, L.O., Kahn, J., Bonnie, R.J., Kass, N.E., Mastroianni, A.C., Moreno, J.D. and Nieburg, P. 2002: Public health ethics: mapping the terrain. *Journal of Law, Medicine and Ethics*, 30 (2), 170–8.

Choi, B.C. 1993: Sensitivity and specificity of a single diagnostic test in the presence of work-up bias. *Journal of Clinical Epidemiology*, 45 (6), 581–6.

Christie, T., Groarke, L. and Sweet, W. 2008: Virtue ethics as an alternative to deontological and consequential reasoning in the harm reduction debate. *International Journal of Drug Policy*, 19, 52–8.

Clarke, A. 1991: Is non-directive genetic counselling possible? *The Lancet*, 338 (8773), 998–1001.

Clarke, A. 1998: Genetic counselling. In R. Chadwick (editor-in-chief) *Encyclopedia of Applied Ethics*, Vol. 2. San Diego: Academic Press, 391–405.

Cochrane, A.L. and Holland, W.W. 1971: Validation of screening procedures. *British Medical Bulletin*, 27 (1), 3–8.

Coker, R. 2004: Compulsory screening of immigrants for tuberculosis and HIV. *British Medical Journal*, 328 (7435), 298–300.

Cole, P. 1995: The moral bases for public health interventions. *Epidemiology*, 6 (1), 78–83.

Coughlin, S.S. 1996a: Model curricula in public health ethics. *American Journal of Preventive Medicine*, 12 (4), 247–51.

Coughlin, S.S. 1996b: Advancing professional ethics in epidemiology. *Journal of Epidemiology and Biostatistics*, 1 (2), 71–7.

Coughlin, S.S. 1996c: Ethically optimized study designs in epidemiology. In S.S. Coughlin and T.L. Beauchamp (eds) *Ethics and Epidemiology*. Oxford: Oxford University Press, 145–55.

Coughlin, S.S. 2000: Ethics and epidemiology at the end of the twentieth century: ethics, values, and mission statements. *Epidemiologic Reviews*, 22 (11), 169–75.

Coughlin, S.S. 2006: Ethical issues in epidemiologic research and public health practice. *Emerging Themes in Epidemiology*, 3 (16), doi:10.1186/1742-7622-3-16.

Coughlin, S.S. and Beauchamp, T.L. (eds) 1996a: *Ethics and Epidemiology*. Oxford: Oxford University Press.

Coughlin, S.S. and Beauchamp, T.L., 1996b: Historical foundations. In S.S. Coughlin and T.L. Beauchamp (eds) *Ethics and Epidemiology*. Oxford: Oxford University Press, 5–23.

Coughlin, S.S. and Etheridge, G.D. 1995: Teaching ethics and epidemiology: initial experiences at two schools of public health. *Epidemiology Monitor*, 16, 5–7.

Coughlin, S.S., Katz, W.H. and Mattison, D.R. 1999: Ethics instruction at schools of public health in the United States. Association of Schools of Public Health Education Committee. *American Journal of Public Health*, 89 (5), 768–70.

Coughlin, S.S., Soskolne, C.L. and Goodman, K.W. 1997: *Case Studies in Public Health Ethics*. Washington, DC: American Public Health Association.

Council for International Organizations of Medical Sciences 2009: *International Ethical Guidelines on Epidemiological Studies*. Geneva: CIOMS.

Council of Ministers of Education, Canada 2003: *Canadian Youth, Sexual Health and HIV/AIDS Study: Factors influencing knowledge, attitudes and behaviours*. Toronto, Ontario: Council of Ministers of Education, Canada. Available at http://www.cmec.ca/Publications/Lists/Publications/Attachments/180/CYSHHAS_2002_EN.pdf (accessed September 2013).

Coveney, J. 1998: The government and ethics of health promotion: the importance of Michel Foucault. *Health Education Research*, 13 (3), 459–68.

Cribb, A. 1995: The borders of health promotion. In D. Seedhouse (ed.) *Reforming Health Care: The Philosophy and Practice of International Health Reform*. Chichester: John Wiley & Sons, 199–207.

Cribb, A. and Dines, A. 1993: What is health promotion? In A. Dines and A. Cribb (eds) *Health Promotion: Concepts and Practice*. Oxford: Blackwell Science, 3–33.

Cribb, A. and Duncan, P. 2002: *Health Promotion and Professional Ethics*. Oxford: Blackwell Science.

D'Amico, R. 1998: Spreading disease: a controversy concerning the metaphysics of disease. *History and Philosophy of the Life Sciences*, 20 (2), 143–62.

Dare, T. 1998: Mass immunisation programmes: some philosophical issues. *Bioethics*, 12 (2), 125–49.

Davis, A., Bamford, J., Wilson, I., Ramkalawan, T., Forshaw, M. and Wright, S. 1997: A critical review of the role of neonatal hearing screening in the detection of congenital hearing impairment. *Health Technology Assessment*, 1 (10), Executive Summary.

Davis, S.K., Winkleby, M.A. and Farquhar, J.W. 1995: Increasing disparity in knowledge of cardiovascular disease risk factors and risk-reduction strategies by socioeconomic status: implications for policymakers. *American Journal of Preventive Medicine*, 11 (5), 318–23.

Dawson, A. 2004: Vaccination and the prevention problem. *Bioethics*, 18 (6), 515–29.

Dawson, A. 2007: Herd protection as a public good: vaccination and our obligations to others. In A. Dawson and M. Verweij (eds) *Ethics, Prevention, and Public Health*. Oxford: Oxford University Press, 160–78.

Delatycki, M.B. 2012: The ethics of screening for disease. *Pathology*, 44 (2), 63–8.

DeMarco, J.P. 2005: Principlism and moral dilemmas: a new principle. *Journal of Medical Ethics*, 31 (2), 101–5.

Department of Health 1998: *Smoking Kills: A White Paper on Tobacco*. London: Stationery Office.

DeVito, S. 2000: On the value-neutrality of the concepts of health and disease: unto the breach again. *The Journal of Medicine and Philosophy*, 25 (5), 539–67.

Diekema, D.S. and the Committee on Bioethics 2005: Responding to parental refusals of immunization of children. *Pediatrics*, 115 (5), 1428–31.

Diekema, D.S. and Marcuse, E.K. 1998: Ethical issues in the vaccination of children. In G.R. Burgio and J.D. Lantos (eds) *Primum Non Nocere Today* (2nd edn). Amsterdam: Elsevier, 37–47.

Donohue-White, P. and Cuddeback, K.F. 2002: The good of health: an argument for an objectivist understanding. In P. Taboada, K.F. Cuddeback and P. Donohue-White (eds) *Person, Society and Value: Towards a Personalist Concept of Health*. Dordrecht: Kluwer, 165–86.

Douard, J.W. 1990: AIDS, stigma, and privacy. *AIDS and Public Policy Journal*, 5 (1), 37–41.

Dougherty, C.J. 1995: Bad faith and victim-blaming: the limits of health promotion. In D. Seedhouse (ed.) *Reforming Health Care: The Philosophy and Practice of International Health Reform*. Chichester: John Wiley & Sons, 209–20.

Downie, R.S. 1990: Ethics in health education: an introduction. In S. Doxiadis (ed.) *Ethics in Health Education*. Chichester: John Wiley & Sons, 3–13.

Doxiadis, S. (ed.) 1990: *Ethics in Health Education*. Chichester: John Wiley & Sons.

Drucker, E. and Clear, A. 1999: Harm reduction in the home of the war on drugs: methadone and needle exchange in the USA. *Drug and Alcohol Review*, 18 (1), 103–12.

Dubé, E., Massé, R. and Noël, L. 2009: Acceptability of harm reduction interventions: contributions of members of the population to the debate about public health ethics. *Canadian Journal of Public Health*, 100 (1), 24–8.

Duncan, P. and Cribb, A. 1996: Helping people change: an ethical approach? *Health Education Research*, 11 (3), 339–48.

Duncan, R.E., Savulescu, J., Gillam, L., Williamson, R. and Delatycki, M.B. 2005: An international survey of predictive genetic testing in children for adult onset conditions. *Genetics in Medicine*, 7 (6), 390–6.

Dworkin, G. 1981: Voluntary health risks and public policy. 1. Taking risks, assessing responsibility. *Hastings Center Report*, 11 (5), 26–31.

Eaves, L.C., Wingert, H. and Ho, H.H. 2006: Screening for autism: agreement with diagnosis. *Autism*, 10 (3), 229–42.

Eavy, G. 2000: Discussion article: Defining illness as action-failure: a response to McKnight. *Journal of Applied Philosophy*, 17 (3), 289–97.

Eide, B.L. 1997: 'The least a parent can do': prenatal genetic testing and the welcome of our children. *Ethics and Medicine*, 13 (3), 59–66.

Elliman, D.A.C., Dezateux, C. and Bedford, H.E. 2002: Newborn and childhood screening programmes: criteria, evidence, and current policy. *Archives of Disease in Childhood*, 87 (1), 6–9.

Elmore, J.G., Barton, M.B., Moceri, V.M., Polk, S., Arena, P.J. and Fletcher, S.W. 1998: Ten-year risk of false positive screening mammograms and clinical breast examinations. *The New England Journal of Medicine*, 338 (16), 1089–96.

Elovich, R. 1996: Staying negative – it's not automatic: a harm-reduction approach to substance use and sex. *AIDS and Public Policy Journal*, 11 (2), 66–77.

Eng, E., Parker, E. and Harlan, C. 1997: Lay health advisor intervention strategies: a continuum from natural helping to paraprofessional helping. *Health Education and Behavior*, 24 (4), 413–17.

Englehardt Jr, H.T. 1975: The concepts of health and disease. In H.T. Englehardt Jr and S.F. Spicker (eds) *Evaluation and Explanation in the Biomedical Sciences*. Dordrecht: Reidel, 125–41.

Englehardt Jr, H.T. 2002: Health, disease and persons: well-being in a postmodern world. In P. Taboada, K.F. Cuddeback and P. Donohue-White (eds) *Person, Society and Value: Towards a Personalist Concept of Health*. Dordrecht: Kluwer, 147–64.

Epstein, C.J. 2000: Some ethical implications of The Human Genome Project. *Genetics in Medicine*, 2 (3), 193–7.

Epstein, R.A. 1997: *Mortal Peril: Our Inalienable Right to Health Care?* Reading, MA: Addison-Wesley.

Etzioni, A. 1993: *The Spirit of Community: Rights, Responsibilities, and the Communitarian Agenda*. New York: Crown Publishers.

Ewles, L. and Simnett, I. 1995: *Promoting Health: A Practical Guide* (3rd edn). London: Scutari.

Faden, R.R. 1987: Ethical issues in government sponsored public health campaigns. *Health Education Quarterly*, 14 (1), 27–37.

Faden, R.R. and Kass, N.E. 1991: Bioethics and public health in the 1980s: resource allocation and AIDS. *Annual Review of Public Health*, 12, 335–60.

Feinberg, J. 1984: *Harm to Others: The Moral Limits of the Criminal Law*. New York: Oxford University Press.

Fost, N. 1992: Ethical implications of screening asymptomatic individuals. *FASEB Journal*, 6 (10), 2813–17.

Fry, C., Treloar, C. and Maher, L. 2007: Applied communitarian ethics for harm reduction: promoting a dialogue within the field. *Drug and Alcohol Review*, 26, 553–5.

Fulford, K.W.M. 1989: *Moral Theory and Medical Practice*. Cambridge: Cambridge University Press.

Fulford, K.W.M. 2001: 'What is (mental) disease?': an open letter to Christopher Boorse. *Journal of Medical Ethics*, 27 (2), 80–5.

Galeotti, A.E. 2007: Relativism, universalism, and applied ethics: the case of female circumcision. *Constellations*, 14 (1), 91–111.

Gauthier, C.C. 2000: Moral responsibility and respect for autonomy: meeting the communitarian challenge. *Kennedy Institute of Ethics Journal*, 10 (4), 337–52.

Gellin, B. 2005: *Misconceptions about Value of Vaccines* (AMA News Brief).

Gillon, R. 1990: Ethics in health promotion and prevention of disease. *Journal of Medical Ethics*, 16 (4), 171–2.

Gillon, R. 1998: Bioethics, Overview. In R. Chadwick (editor-in-chief) *Encyclopedia of Applied Ethics*, Vol. 1. San Diego: Academic Press, 305–17.

Gillott, J. 2001: Screening for disability: a eugenic pursuit? *Journal of Medical Ethics*, 27 (suppl. 2), ii21–3.

Glasziou, P.P., Buchan, H., Del Mar, C., Doust, J., Harris, M., Knight, R., Scott, A., Scott, I.A. and Stockwell, A. 2012: When financial incentives do more good than harm: a checklist. *British Medical Journal*, 345:e5047.

Glover, J. 2001: Future people, disability, and screening. In J. Harris (ed.) *Bioethics*. Oxford: Oxford University Press, 429–44.

Godard, B., Kate, L.T., Evers-Kiebooms, G. and Aymé, S. 2003: Population genetic screening programmes: principles, techniques, practices, and policies. *European Journal of Human Genetics*, 11 (suppl. 2), 549–87.

Goel, V. 2001: Appraising organised screening programmes for testing for genetic susceptibility to cancer. *British Medical Journal*, 322 (7295), 1174–8.

Gold, E.B. 1996: Confidentiality and privacy protection in epidemiologic research. In S.S. Coughlin and T.L. Beauchamp (eds) *Ethics and Epidemiology*. Oxford: Oxford University Press, 128–41.

Goodman, K.W. and Prineas, R.J. 1996: Toward an ethics curriculum in epidemiology. In S.S. Coughlin and T.L. Beauchamp (eds) *Ethics and Epidemiology*. Oxford: Oxford University Press, 290–303.

Gordis, L., Gold, E. and Seltser, R. 1977: Privacy protection in epidemiologic and medical research: a challenge and a responsibility. *American Journal of Epidemiology*, 105 (3), 163–8.

Gostin, L.O. 2000: *Public Health Law: Power, Duty, Restraint*. Berkeley, CA: University of California Press and the Milbank Memorial Fund.

Gostin, L.O. (ed.) 2002a: *Public Health Law and Ethics: A Reader*. Berkeley, CA: University of California Press and the Milbank Memorial Fund.

Gostin, L.O. 2002b: Public health law in an age of terrorism: rethinking individual rights and common goods. *Health Affairs*, 21 (66), 79–93.

Gostin, L.O. 2003: When terrorism threatens health: how far are limitations on personal and economic liberties justified? *Florida Law Review*, 55 (5), 1105–69.

Gostin, L.O. and Lazzarini, Z. 1997: *Human Rights and Public Health in the AIDS Pandemic*. Oxford: Oxford University Press.

Gray, J.A.M. 2004: New concepts in screening. *British Journal of General Practice*, 54 (501), 292–8.

Greenland, S. 1988: Probability versus Popper: an elaboration of the insufficiency of current Popperian approaches for epidemiologic analysis. In K.J. Rothman (ed.) *Causal Inference*. Chestnut Hill, MA: Epidemiology Resources, 95–104.

Greenough, P. 1995: Intimidation, coercion and resistance in the final stages of the South Asian smallpox eradication campaign, 1973–1975. *Social Science and Medicine*, 41 (5), 633–45.

Grier, S. and Bryant, C.A. 2005: Social marketing in public health. *Annual Review of Public Health*, 26, 319–39.

Grimes, D.A. and Schultz, K.F. 2002: Uses and abuses of screening tests. *The Lancet*, 359 (9337), 881–4.

Gruskin, S. and Loff, B. 2002: Do human rights have a role in public health work? *The Lancet*, 360 (9348), 1880.

Guldberg, H. 2000: Child protection and the precautionary principle. In J. Morris (ed.) *Rethinking Risk and the Precautionary Principle*. Oxford: Butterworth-Heinemann, 127–39.

Guttman, N. 2000: *Public Health Communication Interventions: Values and Ethical Dilemmas*. Thousand Oaks, CA: Sage.

Guttman, N. and Salmon, C.T. 2004: Guilt, fear, stigma and knowledge gaps: ethical issues in public health communication interventions. *Bioethics*, 18 (6), 531–52.

Haldane, J. 2005: Free-riders. In T. Honderich (ed.) *The Oxford Companion to Philosophy* (new edn). Oxford: Oxford University Press, 316.

Hall, S. 1992: Should public health respect autonomy? *Journal of Medical Ethics*, 18 (4), 197–201.

Hall, W. 2012: *Harm Reduction Guide to Coming Off Psychiatric Drugs* (2nd edn). Published by The Icarus Project and Freedom Center, available at http://www.theicarusproject.net/downloads/ComingOffPsychDrugsHarmReductGuide2EdZinePrint.pdf (accessed September 2013).

Halpern, S.D., Madison, K.M. and Volpp, K.G. 2009: Patients as mercenaries? The ethics of using financial incentives in the war on unhealthy behaviors. *Circulation: Cardiovascular Quality and Outcomes*, 2 (5), 514–16.

Hare, R.M. 1986: Health. *Journal of Medical Ethics*, 12 (4), 174–81.

Harris, J. and Holm, S. 1995: Is there a moral obligation not to infect others? *British Medical Journal*, 311 (7014), 1215–17.

Hastings, G., MacFadyen, L., Biener, L. and Taylor, T.M. 2002: Debate: Controversies in tobacco control. *Tobacco Control*, 11 (1), 73–7.

Hathaway, A.D. 2002: From harm reduction to human rights: bringing liberalism back into drug reform debates. *Drug and Alcohol Review*, 21, 397–404.

Häyry, H. 1998: Paternalism. In R. Chadwick (editor-in-chief) *Encyclopedia of Applied Ethics*, Vol. 3. San Diego: Academic Press, 449–57.

Häyry, H. and Häyry, M. 1989: Utilitarianism, human rights and the redistribution of health through preventive medical measures. *Journal of Applied Philosophy*, 6 (1), 43–51.

Heath, J., Braun, M.A. and Brindle, M. 2002: Smokers' rights to coronary artery bypass graft surgery. *Journal of Nursing Administration's Healthcare Law, Ethics, and Regulation*, 4 (2), 32–5.

Hedgecoe, A.M. 2004: Critical bioethics: beyond the social science critique of applied ethics. *Bioethics*, 18 (2), 120–43.

Heginbotham, C. 1999: Return to community. In M. Parker (ed.) *Ethics and Community in the Health Care Professions*. London: Routledge, 47–61.

Heller, T., Heller, D. and Pattison, S. 2001: Ethical debate: Vaccination against mumps, measles, and rubella: is there a case for deepening the debate? *British Medical Journal*, 323 (7317), 838–40.

Henderson, R.E. and Newton, N. 2000: Is a universal school entry hearing screen worthwhile? *Ambulatory Child Health*, 6 (4), 247–52.

Herissone-Kelly, P. 2003: Bioethics in the United Kingdom: genetic screening, disability rights, and the erosion of trust. *Cambridge Quarterly on Healthcare Ethics*, 12 (3), 235–41.

Hesslow, G. 1993: Do we need a concept of disease? *Theoretical Medicine and Bioethics*, 14 (1), 1–14.

Hill, A.B. 1965: The environment and disease: association or causation? *Proceedings of the Royal Society of Medicine*, 58, 295–300.

Hobson-West, P. 2003: Understanding vaccination resistance: moving beyond risk. *Health, Risk and Society*, 5 (3), 273–83.

Holland, S. 2003: *Bioethics: A Philosophical Introduction*. Cambridge: Polity.

Holland, S. 2009: Public health paternalism: a response to Nys. *Public Health Ethics*, 2 (3), 285–93.

Holland, S. 2010a: Public health ethics: what it is and how to do it. In S. Peckham and A. Hann (eds) *Public Health Ethics and Practice*. Cambridge: Polity Press, 33–48.

Holland, S. 2010b: Scepticism about the virtue ethics approach to nursing ethics. *Nursing Philosophy*, 11 (3), 151–8.

Holland, S. 2011: The virtue ethics approach to bioethics. *Bioethics*, 25 (4), 192–201.

Holland, S. (ed.) 2012a: *Arguing about Bioethics*. London: Routledge.

Holland S. 2012b: Furthering the sceptical case against virtue ethics in nursing ethics. *Nursing Philosophy*, 13 (4), 266–75.

Holland, S. 2014: Libertarian paternalism and public health nudges. In M. Freeman, S. Hawkes and B. Bennett (eds) *Law and Global Health (Current Legal Issues Volume 16)*. Oxford: Oxford University Press, 331–53.

Holt, R., Beal, J. and Breach, J. 2000: Ethical considerations in water fluoridation. In P. Bradley and A. Burls (eds) *Ethics in Public and Community Health*. London: Routledge, 159–66.

Holtzman, N.A. and Andrews, L.B. 1997: Ethical and legal issues in genetic epidemiology. *Epidemiologic Reviews*, 19 (1), 163–74.

Hooker, B., Mason, E. and Miller, D.E. (eds) 2000: *Morality, Rules, and Consequences*. Edinburgh: Edinburgh University Press.

Hope, T. 2004: *Medical Ethics: A Very Short Introduction*. Oxford: Oxford University Press.

Horner, J.S. 1992: Medical ethics and the public health. *Public Health*, 106 (3), 185–92.

Horner, J.S. 1998: Ethics and the public health. In R. Chadwick and M. Levitt (eds) *Ethical Issues in Community Health Care*. London: Arnold, 34–50.

Horner, J.S. 2000: For debate. The virtuous public health physician. *Journal of Public Health Medicine*, 22 (1), 48–53.

Hyder, A.A. 2000: Ethics and schools of public health. *American Journal of Public Health*, 90 (4), 639–40.

International Epidemiological Association's European Federation 2007: *Good Epidemiological Practice (GEP). Proper Conduct in Epidemiologic Research.* Available at http://ieaweb.org/good-epidemiological-practice-gep/ (accessed March 2014).

International Union for Health Promotion and Education 1999: *The Evidence of Health Promotion Effectiveness: Shaping Public Health in a New Europe.* Brussels: International Union for Health Promotion and Education.

Isaacs, D., Kilham, H.A. and Marshall, H. 2004: Should routine childhood immunizations be compulsory? *Journal of Paediatrics and Child Health*, 40 (7), 392–6.

Jaeschke, R., Guyatt, G. and Sackett, D.L. 1994a: Users' guides to the medical literature. III. How to use an article about a diagnostic test. A. Are the results of the study valid? The Evidence-Based Medicine Working Group. *Journal of the American Medical Association*, 271 (5), 389–91.

Jaeschke, R., Guyatt, G. and Sackett, D.L. 1994b: Users' guides to the medical literature. III. How to use an article about a diagnostic test. B. What are the results and will they help me in caring for my patients? The Evidence-Based Medicine Working Group. *Journal of the American Medical Association*, 271 (9), 703–7.

Jennings, B. 2003: Frameworks for ethics in public health. *Acta Bioethica*, 9 (2), 165–76.

Jepson, R.G., Hewison, J., Thompson, A.G.H. and Weller, D. 2005: How should we measure informed choice? The case of cancer screening. *Journal of Medical Ethics*, 31 (4), 192–6.

Jochelson, K. 2007: *Paying the Patient: Improving Health Using Financial Incentives*. London: King's Fund.

Johannesen, R.L. 1996: *Ethics in Human Communication* (4th edn). Prospect Heights, IL: Waveland Press.

Jones, L., Sidell, M. and Douglas J. (eds) 1997: *The Challenge of Promoting Health: Exploration and Action*. Basingstoke: Macmillan/Open University.

Jonsen, A.R. 1998: *The Birth of Bioethics*. Oxford: Oxford University Press.

Juth, N. and Munthe, C. 2012: *The Ethics of Screening in Health Care and Medicine. Serving Society or Serving the Patient? International Library of Ethics, Law, and the New Medicine*, Vol. 51. Berlin: Springer.

Kass, N.E. 2001: An ethics framework for public health. *American Journal of Public Health*, 91 (11), 1776–82.

Kass, N.E. 2004: Public health ethics: from foundations and frameworks to justice and global public health. *Journal of Law, Medicine and Ethics*, 32 (2), 232–42.

Katz, J. and Peberdy, A. (eds) 1997: *Promoting Health: Knowledge and Practice*. Basingstoke: Macmillan/Open University.

Kennedy, A.M., Brown, C.J. and Gust, D.A. 2005: Vaccine beliefs of parents who oppose compulsory vaccination. *Public Health Reports*, 120 (3), 252–8.

Kessel, A.S. 2003: Public health ethics: teaching survey and critical review. *Social Science and Medicine*, 56 (7), 1439–45.

Khoury, M.J., Beaty, T.H. and Cohen, B.H. 1993: *Fundamentals of Genetic Epidemiology*. Oxford: Oxford University Press.

Khoury, M.J., McCabe, L.L. and McCabe, E.R. 2003: Population screening in the age of genomic medicine. *The New England Journal of Medicine*, 348 (1), 50–8.

Khoury, M.J., Thrasher, J.F., Burke, W., Gettig, E.A., Fridinger, F. and Jackson R. 2000: Challenges in communicating genetics: a public health approach. *Genetics in Medicine*, 2 (3), 198–202.

Khushf, G. 1997: Why bioethics needs the philosophy of medicine: some implications of reflection on concepts of health and disease. *Theoretical Medicine*, 18, 145–63.

King, S. 1999: Vaccination policies: individual rights v community health. *British Medical Journal*, 319 (7223), 1448–9.

Kizer, K.W. 1991: Guidelines for community-based screening for chronic health conditions. *American Journal of Preventive Medicine*, 7 (2), 117–20.

Kleinig, J. 2008: The ethics of harm reduction. *Substance Use and Misuse*, 43 (1), 1–16.

Klugman, C. 2002: Focusing on principles of public health ethics. Presentation at the 130th Annual Meeting of American Public Health Association, November 2002 (Abstract #42837).

Kovács, J. 1998: The concept of disease. *Medicine, Health Care and Philosophy*, 1, 31–9.

Krantz, I., Sachs, L. and Nilstun, T. 2004: Ethics and vaccination. *Scandinavian Journal of Public Health*, 32 (3), 172–8.

Krieger, N. 1994: Epidemiology and the web of causation: has anyone seen the spider? *Social Science and Medicine*, 39 (7), 887–903.

Krieger, N. 1999: Questioning epidemiology: objectivity, advocacy, and socially responsible science. *American Journal of Public Health*, 89 (8), 1151–3.

Krieger, N. and Zierler, S. 1996: What explains the public's health? – A call for epidemiologic theory. *Epidemiology*, 7 (1), 107–9.

Kymlicka, W. 1990: *Contemporary Political Philosophy: An Introduction.* Oxford: Clarendon Press.

Kymlicka, W. 1993: Community. In R.E. Goodin and P. Pettit (eds) *A Companion to Contemporary Political Philosophy.* Oxford: Blackwell Publishers, 366–78.

Lachmann, P.J. 1998: Public health and bioethics. *The Journal of Medicine and Philosophy*, 23 (3), 297–302.

Lalonde, M. (1974). *A New Perspective on the Health of Canadians.* Ottawa: Government of Canada.

Lane, S.D., Rubinstein, R.A., Cibula, D. and Webster, N. 2000: Towards a public health approach to bioethics. *Annals of the New York Academy of Sciences*, 925, 25–36.

Langdridge, D. 2000: The welfare of the child: problems of indeterminacy and deontology. *Human Reproduction*, 15 (3), 502–4.

Lappé, M. 1983: Values and public health: value considerations in setting health policy. *Theoretical Medicine and Bioethics*, 4 (1), 71–92.

Lappé, M. 1985: Virtue and public health: societal obligation and individual need. In E.E. Shelp (ed.) *Virtue and Medicine: Explorations in the Character of Medicine.* Boston, MA: Reidel, 289–303.

Lappé, M. 1986: Ethics and public health. In J.M. Last (ed.) *Maxcy-Rosenau's Public Health and Preventive Medicine* (12th edn). Norwalk, CT: Appleton-Century-Crofts, 1867–77.

Largent, M.A. 2012: *Vaccine: The Debate in Modern America.* Baltimore, MD: Johns Hopkins University Press.

Larson, U. and Okonofua, F.E. 2002: Female circumcision and obstetric complications. *International Journal of Gynecology and Obstetrics*, 77 (3), 255–65.

Last, J.M. 1990: Guidelines on ethics for epidemiologists. *International Journal of Epidemiology*, 19 (1), 226–9.

Last, J.M. 1996: Professional standards of conduct for epidemiologists. In S.S. Coughlin and T.L. Beauchamp (eds) *Ethics and Epidemiology.* Oxford: Oxford University Press, 53–75.

Lavados, M. 2002: Empirical and philosophical aspects of a definition of health and disease. In P. Taboada, K.F. Cuddeback and P. Donohue-White (eds) *Person, Society and Value: Towards a Personalist Concept of Health.* Dordrecht: Kluwer, 187–208.

Le Grand, J. and Srivastava, D. (2009) *Incentives for Prevention: Health England Report No. 3.* Oxford: Health England.

Leeder, S.R. 2004: Ethics and public health. *Internal Medicine Journal*, 34 (7), 435–9.

Leichter, H.M. 1991: *Free to be Foolish: Politics and Health Promotion in the United States and Great Britain.* Princeton, NJ: Princeton University Press.

Lennox, J.G. 1995: Health as an objective value. *The Journal of Medicine and Philosophy*, 20 (5), 499–511.

Lenton, S. and Single, E. 1998: The definition of harm reduction. *Drug and Alcohol Review*, 17, 213–20.

Lenzer, J. 2004: Bush plans to screen whole US population for mental illness. *British Medical Journal*, 328 (7454), 1458.

Leon, D. and Walt, G. (eds) 2001: *Poverty, Inequality and Health: An International Perspective*. Oxford: Oxford University Press.

Leslie, K.M. 2008: Harm reduction: An approach to reducing risky health behaviours in adolescents. *Paediatrics and Child Health*, 13 (1), 53–6.

Levin, B.W. and Fleischman, A.R. 2002: Public health and bioethics: the benefits of collaboration. *American Journal of Public Health*, 92 (2), 165–7.

Levine, C. and Bayer, R. 1985: Screening blood: public health and medical uncertainty. *Hastings Center Report*, 15 (suppl.), 8–11.

Ling, J.C., Franklin, B.A., Lindsteadt, J.F. and Gearon, S.A. 1992: Social marketing: its place in public health. *Annual Review of Public Health*, 13, 341–62.

Lippman, A. 1991: Prenatal genetic testing and screening: constructing needs and reinforcing inequities. *American Journal of Law and Medicine*, 17 (1–2), 15–50.

Loff, B. 2006: Ethical challenges and responses in harm reduction research: a critique of applied communitarian ethics. *Drug and Alcohol Review*, 25, 371–2.

Lorenzi, P. 2004: Sin taxes. *Society*, 41 (3), 59–65.

Lunze, K. and Paasche-Orlow, M.K. 2013: Financial incentives for healthy behavior: ethical safeguards for behavioral economics. *American Journal of Preventive Medicine*, 44 (6), 659–65.

Lyren, A. and Leonard, E. 2006: Vaccine refusal: issues for the primary care physician. *Clinical Pediatrics*, 45 (5), 399–404.

MacDonald, M.A. 2002: Health promotion: historical, philosophical, and theoretical perspectives. In L.E. Young and V. Hayes (eds) *Transforming Health Promotion Practice: Concepts, Issues, and Applications*. Philadelphia, PA: F.A. Davis Co., 22–45.

Mackie, G. 2003: Female genital cutting: a harmless practice? *Medical Anthropology Quarterly*, 17 (2), 135–58.

Mackie, J.L. 1974: *The Cement of the Universe: A Study of Causation*. Oxford: Clarendon Press.

Macklin, R. 2003: Applying the four principles. *Journal of Medical Ethics*, 29 (5), 275–80.

Magnusson, R.S. 2004: 'Underground euthanasia' and the harm minimization debate. *The Journal of Law, Medicine & Ethics*, 32 (3), 486–95.

Maliphant, J. and Scott, J. 2005: Use of the femoral vein ('groin injecting') by a sample of needle exchange clients in Bristol, UK. *Harm Reduction Journal*, 21 (1), 6.

Mann, J. 1995: Human rights and the new public health. *Health and Human Rights*, 1 (3), 229–33.

Marantz, P.R. 1990: Blaming the victim: the negative consequence of preventive medicine. *American Journal of Public Health*, 80 (10), 1186–7.

Marlatt, G.A., Larimer, M.E. and Witkiewitz, K. (eds) 2012: *Harm Reduction: Pragmatic Strategies for Managing High-Risk Behaviours* (2nd edn). New York: The Guilford Press.

Marshall, T. 2000: Exploring a fiscal food policy: the case of diet and ischaemic heart disease. *British Medical Journal*, 320 (7230), 301–5.

Marteau, T., Ashcroft, R. and Oliver, A. 2009: Using financial incentives to achieve healthy behaviour. *British Medical Journal*, 25 (338), 983–5.

Marteau, T.M., Ogilvie, D., Roland, M., Suhrcke, M. and Kelly, M. 2011: Judging nudging: can nudging improve population health? *British Medical Journal*, 342, 263–5.

Martin, R. 2004: Public health ethics and SARS: seeking an ethical framework to global public health governance. *Law, Social Justice and Global Development*, 1 (e-journal).

Massie, R.J., Delatycki, M.B. and Bankier, A. 2005: Screening couples for cystic fibrosis carrier status: why are we waiting? *The Medical Journal of Australia*, 183 (10), 501–2.

May, T. 2005: Public communication, risk perception, and the viability of preventive vaccination against communicable diseases. *Bioethics*, 19 (4), 407–21.

May, T. and Silverman, R.D. 2005: Free-riding, fairness and the rights of minority groups in exemption from mandatory childhood vaccination. *Human Vaccines*, 1 (1), 12–15.

McCloskey, H.J. 1965: A non-utilitarian approach to punishment. *Inquiry*, 8, 239–55.

McCormick, J. 1994: Health promotion: the ethical dimension. *The Lancet*, 344 (8919), 390–1.

McCormick, J. 1996: Medical hubris and the public health. *Journal of Clinical Epidemiology*, 49 (6), 619–21.

McIntyre, P.B., Williams, A.H. and Leask, J.E. 2003: Refusal of parents to vaccinate: dereliction of duty or legitimate personal choice? *The Medical Journal of Australia*, 178 (4), 150–1.

McKeown, R.E. 2000: American College of Epidemiology Ethics Guidelines – filling a critical gap in the profession. *Annals of Epidemiology*, 10 (8), 485–6.

McKeown, R.E., Weed, D.L., Kahn, J.P. and Stoto, M.A. 2003: American College of Epidemiology Ethics Guidelines: Foundations and dissemination. *Science and Engineering Ethics*, 9 (2), 207–14.

McKinnon, W.C., Baty, B.J., Bennett, R.L., Magee, M., Neufeld-Kaiser, W.A., Peters, K.F., Sawyer, J.C. and Schneider, K.A. 1997: Predisposition genetic testing for late-onset disorders in adults. A position paper of the National Society of Genetic Counselors. *Journal of the American Medical Association*, 278 (15), 1217–20.

McKnight, C. 1998: On defining illness. *Journal of Applied Philosophy*, 15 (2), 195–8.

McMullin, E. 1995: Underdetermination. *The Journal of Medicine and Philosophy*, 20 (3), 233–52.

McNally, R.J. 2001: On Wakefield's harmful dysfunction analysis of mental disorder. *Behaviour Research and Therapy*, 39 (3), 309–14.

Megone, C. 1998: Aristotle's function argument and the concept of mental illness. *Philosophy, Psychiatry, and Psychology*, 5 (3), 187–202.

Ménard, J-F 2010: A 'nudge' for public health ethics: libertarian paternalism as a framework for ethical analysis of public health interventions? *Public Health Ethics*, 3 (3), 229–38.

Menzel, P. 1995: Paper four: Non-compliance: fair or free-riding. *Health Care Analysis*, 3 (2), 113–15.

Menzel, P. 2002: Justice and the basic structure of health-care systems. In R. Rhodes, M.P. Battin and A. Silvers (eds) *Medicine and Social Justice: Essays on the Distribution of Health Care*. Oxford: Oxford University Press, 24–37.

Mepham, B. 2005: *Bioethics: An Introduction for the Biosciences*. Oxford: Oxford University Press.

Michels, K.B. 2005: A maternalistic approach to prevention. *International Journal of Epidemiology*, 34 (1), 3–4.

Michie, S., Allanson, A., Armstrong, D., Weinman, J., Bobrow, M. and Marteau, T.M. 1998: Objectives of genetic counselling: differing views of purchasers, providers and users. *Journal of Public Health Medicine*, 20 (4), 404–8.

Mill, J.S. 1950: *Philosophy of Scientific Method*. New York: Hafner.

Mill, J.S. 1975: On liberty. In *Three Essays: On Liberty, Representative Government, The Subjection of Women*. Oxford: Oxford University Press, 5–141.

Miller, P.G., Lintzeris, N. and Forzisi, L. 2008: Is groin injecting an ethical boundary for harm reduction? *International Journal of Drug Policy*, 19 (6), 486–91.

Mitchell, G. 2005: Review essay: Libertarian paternalism is an oxymoron. *Northwestern University Law Review*, 99 (3), 1245–77.

Morgan, O., Meltzer, M., Muir, D., Hogan, H., Seng, C., Hill, J. and Beckford, J. 2003: Specialist vaccination advice and pockets of resistance to MMR vaccination: lessons from an outbreak of measles. *Communicable Disease and Public Health*, 6 (4), 330–3.

Morris, J. 2000. Defining the precautionary principle. In J. Morris (ed.) *Rethinking Risk and the Precautionary Principle*. Oxford: Butterworth-Heinemann, 1–21.

Munthe, C. 2001: Divisibility and the moral status of embryos. *Bioethics*, 15 (5–6), 382–97.

Naidoo, J. and Wills, J. 2000: *Health Promotion: Foundations for Practice* (2nd edn). Edinburgh: Baillière Tindall.

National Screening Committee 1998: *First Report of the National Screening Committee*. London: Health Departments of the United Kingdom.

National Screening Committee 2002: *Antenatal Screening Service for Down's Syndrome in England: 2001. A Report to the UK National Screening Committee.* Oxford: UK National Screening Committee.

Nelson, K.B., Grether, J.K., Croen, L.A., Dambrosia, J.M., Phillips, T.M., Dickens, B.F., Jelliffe, L.L. and Hansen, R.L. 2001: Neuropeptides and neurotrophins in neonatal blood of children with autism or mental retardation. *Annals of Neurology*, 49 (5), 597–606.

Nelson, M.C. and Rogers, J. 1992: The right to die? Anti-vaccination activity and the 1874 smallpox epidemic in Stockholm. *Social History of Medicine*, 5 (3), 369–88.

Newcombe, R. 1992: The reduction of drug related harm: a conceptual framework for theory, practice and research. In P.A. O'Hare, R. Newcombe, A. Matthews, E.C. Buning and E. Drucker (eds) *The Reduction of Drug-Related Harm*. London: Routledge, 1–14.

Nijhuis, H.G.J. and van der Maesen, L.J.G. 1994: The philosophical foundations of public health: an invitation to debate. *Journal of Epidemiology and Community Health*, 48 (1), 1–3.

Nikku, N. 1997: *Informative Paternalism: Studies in the Ethics of Promoting and Predicting Health*. Linköping, Sweden: Linköping Studies in Arts and Science.

Nissen, L. 1993: Four ways of eliminating mind from teleology. *Studies in the History and Philosophy of Science*, 24 (1), 27–48.

Noah, N.D. 1987: Immunisation before school entry: should there be a law? *British Medical Journal*, 294 (6582), 1270–1.

Nordenfelt, L. 1987: *On the Nature of Health: An Action-Theoretic Approach.* Boston, MA: Reidel.

Nordenfelt, L. 1995: On the nature and ethics of health promotion: an attempt at a systematic analysis. In D. Seedhouse (ed.) *Reforming Health Care: The Philosophy and Practice of International Health Reform*. Chichester: John Wiley & Sons, 185–207.

Nordenfelt, L. 2003: On the evolutionary concept of health: health as natural function. In L. Nordenfelt and P.-E. Liss (eds) *Dimensions of Health and Health Promotion*. Amsterdam: Rodopi, 37–54.

Norman, R.J. 2005: Autonomy in applied ethics. In T. Honderich (ed.) *The Oxford Companion to Philosophy* (new edition). Oxford: Oxford University Press, 72.

Nuffield Council on Bioethics 1993: *Genetic Screening: Ethical Issues*. London: Nuffield Council on Bioethics.

Nuffield Council on Bioethics 2007: *Public Health: Ethical Issues*. London: Nuffield Council on Bioethics.

O'Hagan, J. 1991: The ethics of informed consent in relation to prevention screening programmes. *The New Zealand Medical Journal*, 104 (908), 121–3.

O'Neill, O. 2002: Public health or clinical ethics: thinking beyond borders. *Ethics and International Affairs*, 16 (2), 35–45.

O'Riordan, T. and Cameron, J. (eds) 1994: *Interpreting the Precautionary Principle*. London: Earthscan.

O'Riordan, T., Cameron, J. and Jordan, A. (eds) 2001: *Reinterpreting the Precautionary Principle*. London: Cameron May.

Oliver, A. 2012: A nudge too far? A nudge at all? On paying people to be healthy. *Healthcare Papers*, 12 (4), 8–16.

Ottawa Charter for Health Promotion 1986: *Health Promotion International*, 1 (4), 405.

Parascandola, M. and Weed, D.L. 2001: Causation in epidemiology. *Journal of Epidemiology and Community Health*, 55 (12), 905–12.

Parens, E. and Asch, A. 1999: The disability rights critique of prenatal genetic testing: reflections and recommendations. *Hastings Center Report*, 29 (5) (special suppl.), S1–22.

Parens, E. and Asch, A. (eds) 2000: *Prenatal Testing and Disability Rights*. Washington, DC: Georgetown University Press.

Parker, J. 1998: Precautionary principle. In R. Chadwick (editor-in-chief) *Encyclopedia of Applied Ethics*, Vol. 3. San Diego, CA: Academic Press, 633–41.

Parker, L.S. 1995: Breast cancer genetic screening and critical bioethics' gaze. *The Journal of Medicine and Philosophy*, 20 (3), 313–37.

Parker, M. 1996: Communitarianism and its problems. *Cogito*, 10 (3), 204–9.

Parker, M. 1998: Individualism. In R. Chadwick and M. Levitt (eds) *Ethical Issues in Community Health Care*. London: Arnold, 16–23.

Parmet, W. 2003: Liberalism, communitarianism, and public health: comments on Lawrence O. Gostin's lecture. *Florida Law Review*, 55 (5), 1221–40.

Pellegrino, E.D. 1995: Guarding the integrity of medical ethics: some lessons from Soviet Russia. *The Journal of the American Medical Association*, 273 (20), 1622–3.

Plotkin, S.L. and Plotkin, S.A. 1994: A short history of vaccination. In S.A. Plotkin and E.A. Mortimer (eds.) *Vaccines* (2nd edn). Philadelphia, PA: W.B. Saunders, 1–11.

Public Health Leadership Society 2002: *Principles of the Ethical Practice of Public Health*. Public Health Leadership Society. Available at http://www.apha.org/NR/rdonlyres/1CED3CEA-287E-4185-9CBD-BD405FC60856/0/ethicsbrochure.pdf (accessed March 2014).

Pywell, S. 2000: Vaccination and other altruistic medical treatments: should autonomy or communitarianism prevail? *Medical Law International*, 4 (3–4), 223–43.

Rachels, J. and Rachels, S. 2007: *The Elements of Moral Philosophy* (5th edn). Boston, MA: McGraw-Hill.

Raeder, L.C. 1998: Liberalism and the common good: a Hayekian perspective on communitarianism. *Independent Review*, 2 (4), 519–35.

Rahi, J.S., Williams, C., Bedford, H. and Elliman, D. 2001: Screening and surveillance for ophthalmic disorders and visual deficits in children in the United Kingdom. *British Journal of Ophthalmology*, 85 (3), 257–9.

Räikkä, J. 1996: The social concept of disease. *Theoretical Medicine*, 17, 353–61.

Ramsay, J., Richardson, J., Carter, Y.H., Davidson, L.L. and Feder, G. 2002: Should health professionals screen women for domestic violence? Systematic review. *British Medical Journal*, 325 (7539), 314–18.

Renton, A. 1994: Epidemiology and causation: a realist view. *Journal of Epidemiology and Community Health*, 48 (1), 79–85.

Reymond, L., Mohamud, A. and Nancy, A. 1997: Female genital mutilation – the facts. Program for Appropriate Technology in Health. Available at http://www.path.org/publications/files/path_the_facts_fgm.pdf (accessed September 2013).

Reynolds, T.M. 2003: Down's syndrome screening is unethical: views of today's research ethics committees. *Journal of Clinical Pathology*, 56 (4), 268–70.

Reznek, L. 1987: *The Nature of Disease*. London: Routledge and Kegan Paul.

Rhodes, R. 2006: Why test children for adult-onset genetic diseases? *The Mount Sinai Journal of Medicine*, 73 (3), 609–16.

Rhodes, T. and Hedrich, D. (ed.) 2010: *Harm Reduction: Evidence, Impacts and Challenges (EMCDDA Monographs)*. Luxembourg: Publications Office of the European Union.

Rhodes, T., Stoneman, A., Hope, V., Hunt, N., Martin, A. and Judd, A. 2006: Groin injecting in the context of crack cocaine and homelessness: From 'risk boundary' to 'acceptable risk'? *International Journal of Drug Policy*, 17, 164–70.

Rizzo, M.J. and Whitman, D.G. 2009: Little brother is watching you: new paternalism on the slippery slopes. *Arizona Law Review*, 51 (3), 685–739.

Roberts, M.J.R. and Reich, M.R. 2002: Ethical analysis in public health. *The Lancet*, 359 (9311), 1055–9.

Robins, D.L., Fein, D., Barton, M.L. and Green, J.A. 2001: The modified-checklist for autism in toddlers: an initial study investigating the early detection of autism and pervasive developmental disorders. *Journal of Autism and Developmental Disorders*, 31 (2), 131–44.

Roden, J. 2004: Revisiting the health belief model: nurses applying it to young families and their health promotion needs. *Nursing and Health Sciences*, 6 (1), 1–10.

Rogers, A., Pilgrim, D., Gust, I.D., Stone, D.H. and Menzel, P.T. 1995: Discussion: The pros and cons of immunisation. *Health Care Analysis*, 3 (2), 99–115.

Rosen, A. 2000: Ethics of early prevention in schizophrenia. *Australian and New Zealand Journal of Psychiatry*, 34 (suppl.), S208–12.

Rossignol, A.M. and Goodmonson, S. 1995: Are ethical topics in epidemiology included in the graduate epidemiology curricula? *American Journal of Epidemiology*, 142 (12), 1265–8.

Rothman, K.J. 1976: Causes. *American Journal of Epidemiology*, 104 (6), 587–92.

Rothman, K.J. (ed.) 1988: *Causal Inference*. Chestnut Hill, MA: Epidemiology Resources.

Rothman, K.J. 2002: *Epidemiology: An Introduction*. Oxford: Oxford University Press.

Rothman, K.J. and Greenland, S. (eds) 1998: *Modern Epidemiology* (2nd edn). Philadelphia, PA: Lippincott-Raven.

Rothstein, M.A. 2004: Are traditional public health strategies consistent with contemporary American values? *Temple Law Review*, 77 (2), 175–92.

Rouse, A. and Adab, P. 2001: Is population coronary heart disease risk screening justified? A discussion of the National Service Framework for coronary heart disease (Standard 4). *British Journal of General Practice*, 51 (471), 834–7.

Royal Society of Canada 2001: *Elements of Precaution: Recommendation for the Regulation of Food Biotechnology in Canada*. Ottawa: Royal Society of Canada.

Ruderman, R. 2013: Female circumcision: the ethics of harm reduction policies. *The Michigan Journal of Public Affairs*, 10, 95–107.

Ryan, A. 1993: Liberalism. In R.E. Goodin and P. Pettit (eds) *A Companion to Contemporary Political Philosophy*. Oxford: Blackwell Publishers, 291–311.

Saha, P. 2002: Breastfeeding and sexuality: professional advice literature from the 1970s to the present. *Health Education and Behavior*, 29 (1), 61–72.

Salazar, A.R. 2012: Libertarian paternalism and the danger of nudging consumers. *King's Law Journal*, 23 (1), 51–67.

Salmon, C.T. (ed.) 1989: *Information Campaigns: Balancing Social Values and Social Change*. Newbury Park, CA: Sage.

Salmon, D.A., Haber, M., Gangarosa, E.J., Phillips, L., Smith, N.J. and Chen, R.T. 1999: Health consequences of religious and philosophical exemptions from immunization laws: individual and societal risk of measles. *The Journal of the American Medical Association*, 281 (1), 47–53.

Salmon, D.A., Moulton, L.H., Omer, S.B., DeHart, M.P., Stokley, S. and Halsey, N.A. 2005: Factors associated with refusal of childhood vaccines among parents of school-aged children: a case-control study. *Archives of Pediatrics and Adolescent Medicine*, 159 (5), 470–6.

Sandel, M.J. 1982: *Liberalism and the Limits of Justice*. Cambridge: Cambridge University Press.

Santangelo, S.L. and Tsatsanis, K. 2005: What is known about autism: genes, brains, and behavior. *American Journal of Pharmacogenomics*, 5 (2), 71–92.

Schaffner, K.F. 1999: Coming home to Hume: a sociobiological foundation for a concept of 'health' and morality. *The Journal of Medicine and Philosophy*, 24 (4), 365–75.

Schmidt, T.A. 1995: When public health competes with individual needs. *Academic Emergency Medicine*, 2 (3), 217–22.

Schramm, F.R. and Kottow, M. 2001: Bioethical principles in public health: limitations and proposals. *Cadernos de Saúde Pública*, 17 (4), 949–56.

Seedhouse, D. 1986: *Health: The Foundations for Achievement*. Chichester: John Wiley & Sons.

Seedhouse, D. 1995: 'Well-being': health promotion's red herring. *Health Promotion International*, 10 (1), 61–7.

Seedhouse, D. 2004: *Health Promotion: Philosophy, Prejudice and Practice* (2nd edn). Chichester: John Wiley & Sons.

Seifert, J. and Taboada, P. 2002: Epilogue. In P. Taboada, K.F. Cuddeback and P. Donohue-White (eds) *Person, Society and Value: Towards a Personalist Concept of Health*. Dordrecht: Kluwer, 241–52.

Serra-Prat, M., Gallo, P., Jovell, A.J., Aymerich, M. and Estrada, M.D. 1998: Trade-offs in prenatal detection of Down syndrome. *American Journal of Public Health*, 88 (4), 551–7.

Shefer, A., Briss, P. and Rodewald, L. 1999: Improving immunization coverage rates: an evidence-based review of the literature. *Epidemiologic Reviews*, 21 (1), 96–142.

Shell-Duncan, B. 2001: The medicalization of female 'circumcision': harm reduction or promotion of a dangerous practice? *Social Science & Medicine*, 52, 1013–28.

Shickle, D. and Chadwick, R. 1994: The ethics of screening: is 'screeningitis' an incurable disease? *Journal of Medical Ethics*, 20, 12–18.

Sidel, V.W., Cohen, H.W. and Gould, R.M. 2002: Bioterrorism preparedness: cooptation of public health. *Medicine and Global Survival*, 7 (2), 82–9.

Silverman, M., Terry, M.A., Zimmerman, R.K., Nutini, J.F. and Ricci, E.M. 2002: The role of qualitative methods for investigating barriers to adult immunization. *Qualitative Health Research*, 12 (8), 1058–75.

Sindall, C. 2002: Does health promotion need a code of ethics? *Health Promotion International*, 17 (3), 201–3.

Singleton, J. and McLaren, S. 1995: *Ethical Foundations of Health Care: Responsibilities in Decision Making*. London: Mosby.

Sirico, R.A. 1995: The sin tax: economic and moral considerations. Occasional Paper No. 5. Grand Rapids, MI: Acton Institute for the Study of Religion and Liberty.

Skrabanek, P. 1988: The debate over mass mammography in Britain. The case against. *British Medical Journal*, 297 (6654), 971–2.

Skrabanek, P. 1990: Why is preventive medicine exempted from ethical constraints? *Journal of Medical Ethics*, 16 (4), 187–90.

Sleep, J. 1991: Development of international ethical guidelines for epidemiological research and practice. Report of the proceedings of the 25th Council for the International Organisation of Medical Sciences (CIOMS) conference, WHO headquarters. Geneva, Switzerland, 7–9 November 1990. *Midwifery*, 7 (1), 42–4.

Slevin, E. 2004: High intensity counselling or behavioural interventions can result in moderate weight loss. *Evidence-based Healthcare*, 8 (3), 136–8.

Smart, J.J.C. and Williams, B. 1973: *Utilitarianism: For and Against*. Cambridge: Cambridge University Press.

Smith, D.R. 2000: Immunization in the new millennium: meeting the challenge to realize the promise. *American Journal of Preventive Medicine*, 19 (3S), 1–3.

Smith, P.J., Chu, S.Y. and Barker, L.E. 2004: Children who have received no vaccines: who are they and where do they live? *Pediatrics*, 114 (1), 187–95.

Smith, S.W. 2007: Some realism about end of life: the current prohibition and the euthanasia underground. *American Journal of Law and Medicine*, 33, 55–95.

Society of Health Education and Health Promotion Specialists 2007: *A Framework for Ethical Health Promotion*. Available at www.rsph.org.uk.

Sorell, T. 2007: Parental choice and expert knowledge in the debate about MMR and autism. In A. Dawson and M. Verweij (eds) *Ethics, Prevention, and Public Health*. Oxford: Oxford University Press, 95–110.

Soskolne, C.L. and Light, A. 1996: Towards ethics guidelines for environmental epidemiologists. *The Science of the Total Environment*, 184 (1), 137–47.

Soskolne, C.L. and MacFarlane, D.K. 1996: Scientific misconduct in epidemiologic research. In S.S. Coughlin and T.L. Beauchamp (eds) *Ethics and Epidemiology*. Oxford: Oxford University Press, 274–89.

Sox, H.C. 1998: Benefit and harm associated with screening for breast cancer. *The New England Journal of Medicine*, 338 (16), 1145–6.

Stempsey, W.E. 2000: A pathological view of disease. *Theoretical Medicine and Bioethics*, 21 (4), 321–30.

Stevenson, D. 2006: Libertarian paternalism: the cocaine vaccine as a test case for the Sunstein/Thaler model. *Rutgers University Journal of Law and Urban Policy*, 1 (3), 4–62.

Stewart-Brown, S. 1999: Childhood screening. In P. Bradley and A. Burls (eds) *Ethics in Public and Community Health*. London: Routledge, 119–31.

Stone, D.H. 1995: Paper three: The difference between ideological and intellectual dissent. *Health Care Analysis*, 3 (2), 111–13.

Stone, D.H. and Stewart, S. 1996: Screening and the new genetics; a public health perspective on the ethical debate. *Journal of Public Health and Medicine*, 18 (1), 3–5.

Stone, W.L., Coonrod, E.E. and Ousley, O.Y. 2000: Brief report – screening tool for autism in two-year-olds (STAT): development and preliminary data. *Journal of Autism and Developmental Disorders*, 30 (6), 607–12.

Stone, W.L., Coonrod, E.E., Turner, L.M. and Pozdol, S.L. 2004: Psychometric properties of the STAT for early autism screening. *Journal of Autism and Developmental Disorders*, 34 (6), 691–701.

Streefland, P.H. 2001: Public doubts about vaccination safety and resistance against vaccination. *Health Policy*, 55 (3), 159–72.

Strock, M. 2004: *Autism Spectrum Disorders (Pervasive Developmental Disorders)*. Bethesda, MD: National Institute of Mental Health.

Sullivan, R.J. 1994: *An Introduction to Kant's Ethics*. Cambridge: Cambridge University Press.

Sunstein, C.R. and Thaler, R.H. 2003: Libertarian paternalism is not an oxymoron. *University of Chicago Law Review*, 70 (4), 1159–202.

Supreme Court of Canada 2011: Canada (Attorney General) v. PHS Community Services Society. Available at http://scc.lexum.org/en/2011/2011scc44/2011scc44.html (accessed September 2013).

Susser, M. 1991: What is a cause and how do we know one? A grammar for pragmatic epidemiology. *American Journal of Epidemiology*, 133 (7), 635–48.

Susser, M. and Susser, E. 1996a: Choosing a future for epidemiology. I. Eras and paradigms. *American Journal of Public Health*, 86 (5), 668–73.

Susser, M. and Susser, E. 1996b: Choosing a future for epidemiology. II. From black box to Chinese boxes and eco-epidemiology. *American Journal of Public Health*, 86 (5), 674–7.

Swift, A. 2001: *Political Philosophy: A Beginners' Guide for Students and Politicians*. Cambridge: Polity.

Szasz, T.S. 1960: The myth of mental illness. *American Psychologist*, 15 (2), 113–18.

Szilagyi, P., Vann, J., Bordley, C., Chelminski, A., Kraus, R., Margolis, P. and Rodewald, L. 2002: Interventions aimed at improving immunization rates. *The Cochrane Database of Systematic Reviews*, 4 (CD003941).

Tatara, K. 2002: Philosophy of public health: lessons from its history in England. *Journal of Public Health Medicine*, 24 (1), 11–15.

Thaler, R.H. and Sunstein, C.R. 2003: Libertarian paternalism. *The American Economic Review*, 93 (2), 175–9.

Thaler, R.H. and Sunstein, C.R. 2009: *Nudge: Improving Decisions about Health, Wealth and Happiness* (rev. int. edn). London: Penguin.

Thomas, D.C. 2004: *Statistical Methods in Genetic Epidemiology*. New York: Oxford University Press.

Thomas, J.C. 2003: Teaching ethics in schools of public health. *Public Health Reports*, 118, 279–86.

Thomas, J.C., Sage, M., Dillenberg, J. and Guillory, V.J. 2002: A code of ethics for public health. *American Journal of Public Health*, 92 (7), 1057–9.

Thomasma, D.C. 1997: Antifoundationalism and the possibility of a moral philosophy of medicine. *Theoretical Medicine*, 18 (1–2), 127–43.

Thornton T. 2000: Mental illness and reductionism: can functions be naturalized? *Philosophy, Psychiatry, and Psychology*, 7 (1), 67–76.

Tooley, M. 1972: Abortion and infanticide. *Philosophy and Public Affairs*, 2 (1), 37–65.

Tooley, M. 1980: An irrelevant consideration: killing versus letting die. In B. Steinbock (ed.) *Killing and Letting Die*. New York: Fordham University Press, 56–62.

Tooley, M. 1998: Personhood. In H. Kuhse and P. Singer (eds) *A Companion to Bioethics*. Oxford: Blackwell, 117–26.

Toumbourou, J.W. Stockwell, T., Neighbors, C., Marlatt, G.A., Sturge, J. and Rehm, J. 2007: Interventions to reduce harm associated with adolescent substance use. *Lancet*, 369, 1391–401.

Tountas, Y., Garanis, T.N. and Dalla-Vorgia, P. 1994: Health promotion, society and health care ethics. In R. Gillon (ed.) *Principles of Health Care Ethics*, Chichester: John Wiley & Sons, 843–54.

Turnock, B.J. 2004: *Public Health: What it is and How it Works* (3rd edn). Sudbury, MA: Jones and Bartlett.

UKHRA 2013: Harm reduction defined. Available at http://www.ukhra.org/harm_reduction_definition.html (accessed September 2013).

Underwood, M.J., Bailey, J.S., Shiu, M., Higgs, R. and Garfield, J. 1993: Should smokers be offered coronary bypass surgery? *British Medical Journal*, 306 (6884), 1047–50.

Upshur, R.E. 2002: Principles for the justification of public health intervention. *Canadian Journal of Public Health*, 93 (2), 101–3.

US Department of Health, Education, and Welfare 1979: *Healthy People: The Surgeon General's Report on Health Promotion and Disease Prevention*. Washington, DC: Public Health Service, Office of the Assistant Secretary for Health (DHEW Publication No. (PHS) 7950066).

US Preventive Services Task Force 1996: *Guide to Clinical Preventive Services* (2nd edn). Baltimore, MD: Williams and Wilkins.

US Preventive Services Task Force 2003: Screening for obesity in adults: recommendations and rationale. *Annals of Internal Medicine*, 139 (11), 930–2.

van der Maesen, L.J.G. and Nijhuis, H.G.J. 2000: Continuing the debate on the philosophy of modern public health: social quality as a point of reference. *Journal of Epidemiology and Community Health*, 54 (2), 134–42.

van Spijk, P. 2002: Positive and negative aspects of the WHO definition of health, and their implications for a new concept of health in the future. In P. Taboada, K.F. Cuddeback and P. Donohue-White (eds) *Person, Society and Value: Towards a Personalist Concept of Health*. Dordrecht: Kluwer, 209–28.

Veal, A.J. 1993: The concept of lifestyle: a review. *Leisure Studies*, 12 (4), 233–52.

Veatch, R.M. 1980: Voluntary risks to health: the ethical issues. *The Journal of the American Medical Association*, 243 (1), 50–5.

Veatch, R.M. and Stempsey, W.E. 1995: Incommensurability: its implications for the patient/physician relation. *The Journal of Medicine and Philosophy*, 20 (3), 253–69.

Vernon J.G. 2003: Immunisation policy: from compliance to concordance? *British Journal of General Practice*, 53 (490), 399–404.

Verweij, M. 2005: Obligatory precautions against infection. *Bioethics*, 19 (4), 323–35.

Verweij, M. and Dawson, A. 2004: Ethical principles for collective immunisation programmes. *Vaccine*, 22 (23–24), 3122–6.

Visintainer, C.L., Matthias-Hagen, V. and Nance, M.A. 2001: Anonymous predictive testing for Huntington's disease in the United States. *Genetic Testing*, 5 (3), 213–18.

Vogel, F. and Motulsky, A.G. 2002. Human and medical genetics. In R. Detels, J. McEwen, R. Beaglehole and H. Tanaka (eds) *Oxford Textbook of Public Health* (4th edn). Oxford: Oxford University Press, 131–48.

Wakefield, J.C. 1992a: The concept of mental disorder: on the boundary between biological facts and social values. *American Psychologist*, 47 (3), 373–88.

Wakefield, J.C. 1992b: Disorder as harmful dysfunction: a conceptual critique of DSM-III-R's definition of mental disorder. *Psychological Review*, 99 (2), 232–47.

Wakefield, J.C. 2000: Aristotle as sociobiologist: the 'function of a human being' argument, black box essentialism, and the concept of mental disorder. *Philosophy, Psychiatry, and Psychology*, 7 (1), 17–44.

Walzer, M. 1990: The communitarian critique of liberalism. *Political Theory*, 18 (1), 6–23.

Weed, D.L. 1994: Alcohol, breast cancer, and causal inference: where ethics meets epidemiology. *Contemporary Drug Problems*, 21 (1), 185–204.

Weed, D.L. 1996: Epistemology and ethics in epidemiology. In S.S. Coughlin and T.L. Beauchamp (eds) *Ethics and Epidemiology*. Oxford: Oxford University Press, 76–94.

Weed, D.L. 1997: Underdetermination and incommensurability in contemporary epidemiology. *Kennedy Institute of Ethics Journal*, 7 (2), 107–24.

Weed, D.L. 1999: Towards a philosophy of public health. *Journal of Epidemiology and Community Health*, 53 (2), 99–104.

Weed, D.L. 2002/2003: Is the precautionary principle a principle? *IEEE Technology and Society Magazine*, 21 (4), 45–8.

Weed, D.L. and Coughlin, S.S. 1999: New ethics guidelines for epidemiology: background and rationale. *Annals of Epidemiology*, 9 (5), 277–80.

Weed, D.L. and Gorelic, L.S. 1996: The practice of causal inference in cancer epidemiology. *Cancer Epidemiology Biomarkers and Prevention*, 5 (4), 303–11.

Weed, D.L. and Kramer, B.S. 1996: Induced abortion, bias, and breast cancer: why epidemiology hasn't reached its limit. *Journal of the National Cancer Institute*, 88 (23), 1689–700.

Weed, D.L. and McKeown, R.E. 1998: Epidemiology and virtue ethics. *International Journal of Epidemiology*, 27, 343–9.

Weed, D.L. and McKeown, R.E. 2003: Science and social responsibility in public health. *Environmental Health Perspectives*, 111 (14), 1804–8.

Weed, D.L. and Mink, P.J. 2002: Roles and responsibilities of epidemiologists. *Annals of Epidemiology*, 12 (2), 67–72.

Westrin, C.-G., Nilstun, T., Smedby, B. and Haglund, B. 1992: Epidemiology and moral philosophy. *Journal of Medical Ethics*, 18 (4), 193–6.

Wheeler, D.C., Szymanski, K.M., Black, A. and Nelson, D.E. 2011: Applying strategies from libertarian paternalism to decision making for prostate specific antigen (PSA) screening. *BMC Cancer*, 11, 148.

Whitelaw, S. and Watson, J. 2005: Whither health promotion events? A judicial approach to evidence. *Health Education Research*, 20 (2), 214–25.

Whitelaw, S. and Whitelaw, A. 1996: Response: What do we expect from ethics in health promotion and where does Foucault fit in? *Health Education Research*, 11 (3), 349–54.

Wikler, D. 1978: Persuasion and coercion for health: ethical issues in government efforts to change life-styles. *The Milbank Memorial Fund Quarterly. Health and Society*, 56 (3), 303–8.

Wikler, D. 1997: Presidential address: Bioethics and social responsibility. *Bioethics*, 11 (3–4), 185–92.

Wilkinson, T.M. 2009: Making people be healthy. *Journal of Primary Health Care*, 1 (3), 244–6.

Williams, G. 1984: Health promotion – caring concern or slick salesmanship? *Journal of Medical Ethics*, 10 (4), 191–5.

Wilson, J.M.G. and Jungner, Y.G. 1968: *Principles and Practice of Screening for Disease*. Geneva: World Health Organization.

Wing, S. 1994: Limits of epidemiology. *Medicine and Global Survival*, 1 (2), 74–86.

Witte, K. 1994: The manipulative nature of health communication research: ethical issues and guidelines. *American Behavioral Scientist*, 38 (2), 285–93.

Wodak, A. 2007: Ethics and drug policy. *Psychiatry*, 6 (2), 59–62.

World Health Organization 1948: *Preamble to the Constitution of the World Health Organization*. Geneva: World Health Organization.

Wynder, E.L., Higgins, I.T. and Harris, R.E. 1990: The wish bias. *Journal of Clinical Epidemiology*, 43 (6), 619–21.

Wynia, M.K. 2005a: Public health principlism: the precautionary principle and beyond. *The American Journal of Bioethics*, 5 (3), 3–4.

Wynia, M.K. 2005b: Science, faith and AIDS: the battle over harm reduction. *American Journal of Bioethics*, 5 (2), 3–4.

Yeo, M. 1993: Toward an ethic of empowerment for health promotion. *Health Promotion International*, 8 (3), 225–35.

Zador, D., Lintzeris, N., van der Waal, R., Miller, P., Metrebian, N. and Strang, J. 2008: The fine line between harm reduction and harm production – development of a clinical policy on femoral (groin) injecting. *European Addiction Research*, 14 (4), 213–18.

Zwaigenbaum, L., Bryson, S., Rogers, T., Roberts, W., Brian, J. and Szatmari, P. 2005: Behavioral manifestations of autism in the first year of life. *International Journal of Developmental Neuroscience*, 23 (2–3), 143–52.

Zwart, H. 1999: All you need is health. Liberal and communitarian views on the allocation of health care resources. In M. Parker (ed.) *Ethics and Community in the Health Care Professions*. London: Routledge, 30–46.

Index